SHIATSU

A beginner's guide

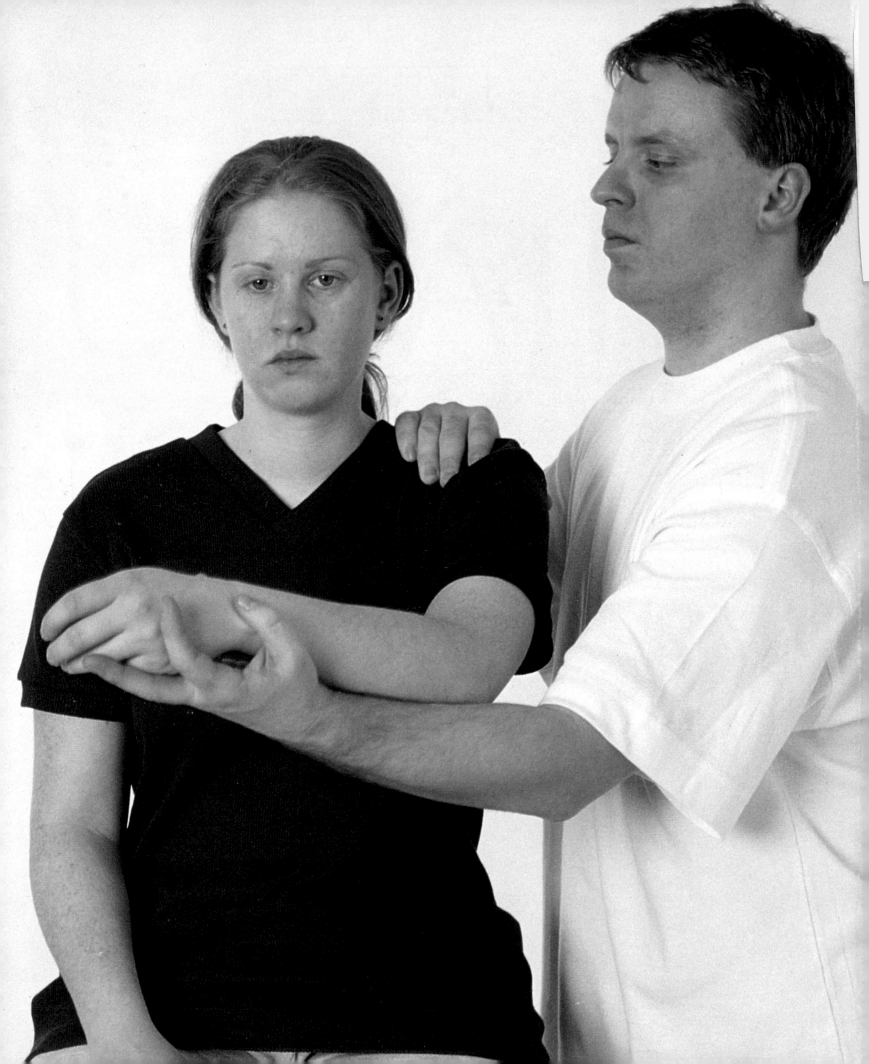

SHIATSU

A
beginner's
guide

Ray Pawlett

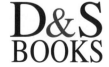

D&S
BOOKS

First published in 2001 by D&S Books

© 2001 D&S Books

D&S Books
Cottage Meadow, Bocombe,
Parkham, Bideford
Devon, England
EX39 5PH

e-mail us at:-
enquiries.dspublishing@care4free.net

This edition printed 2001

ISBN 1-903327-21-0

Editorial director: Sarah King
Editor: Sarah Harris
Project editor: Clare Haworth-Maden
Designer: 2H Design
Photography: Colin Bowling

Distributed in the UK & Ireland by
Bookmart Limited
Desford Road
Enderby
Leicester LE9 5AD

Distributed in Australia by
Herron Books
39 Commercial Road
Fortitude Valley
Queensland 4006

1 3 5 7 9 10 8 6 4 2

This book is in no way intended to replace any qualified medical opinions. If you are ill or in need of treatment, you should consult a qualified doctor or healer. The contents of this book do not qualify any reader to become a healer and any work done is at own risk.

Contents

Introduction

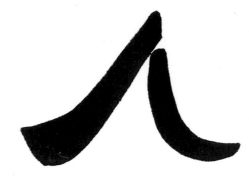

When working with Eastern methods, such as Shiatsu and Tai Chi, I have frequently encountered people who have an interest in the area, but have not, as yet, 'taken the plunge' and become involved. They sometimes have an intuitive grasp of the richness of these areas of knowledge, but hold themselves back from exploring a fascinating world of self-discovery. The reason why they are not giving it a try frequently makes a parallel with exactly why they should be doing it. For example, being 'too busy' is something that you may help yourself to put into perspective if you have a few Shiatsu treatments.

The deep-rooted reason is normally fear of the unknown. One of the aims of this book is to present information in a simple format to help to bridge this gap in understanding. It is therefore aimed at the type of person who may be thinking of starting a Shiatsu treatment or course, but wishes to learn more before committing.

The book will also be useful in the beginning stages of a Shiatsu course. At this stage, most students will be trying to assimilate as much information as possible. It is hoped that this book will provide some easy-to-digest reading that will help the process.

The book is divided into four sections – theory, analysis, practice and reflection – because this is how we learn. You will need to start with some basic knowledge or theory. You will then need to understand how this applies to the person you are working with through analysis and diagnosis. When you have made your diagnosis, you will need to put your knowledge into practice. You then need to reflect on the process so that you can learn from it.

Good luck!

What is Shiatsu?

Anybody who picks up and opens this book will gain an idea of what Shiatsu is. The idea may only come from seeing the pictures on the cover, or it may came from a treatment that you have had earlier. Think for a moment and try to crystallise what you think Shiatsu is. You may prefer to do this as a mental exercise or else write your ideas down. The important thing is to focus on your own definition as it stands at the moment.

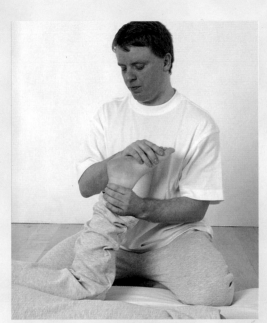

It is easier to learn a subject if you can define what your goals are. The first goal of learning a subject is therefore to define what the subject means to you. For example, if you could ask Einstein, Stephen Hawking and the next person you speak to for their definition of science, you would get a different answer from each. None of them would be wrong; it is simply that we all have different viewpoints.

A common definition of Shiatsu is something like 'acupuncture without needles'. This idea comes from the fact that the Japanese word *Shiatsu* literally translates as 'finger pressure'. The implication here is that finger pressure is used to stimulate the flow of energy in the recipient and thus to assist the healing process.

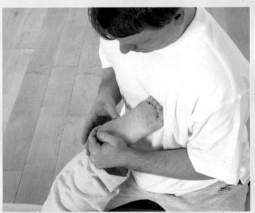

This definition is true, but limited. In Shiatsu, you can also use your hands, feet, elbows, forearms and knees. You may be holding, pressing, stretching, twisting or rocking the recipient.

To do this efficiently, you will need to develop sensitivity and poise. If you cannot feel the changes, you will have no idea of where your treatment is leading you. If you cannot move smoothly when practising Shiatsu, the energy flow is impaired.

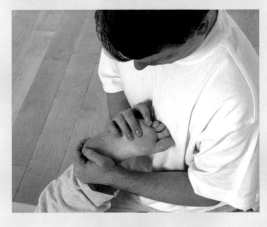

You will also need to develop your own energy, or Ki. How can you cause changes in somebody else if you cannot change yourself? Sensitivity, balance and energy will not happen if you are not grounded. If your grounding is good, then you stand a better chance of helping somebody.

The qualities that you will develop through learning Shiatsu will not stop there. For example, how can you treat without empathy? Shiatsu is a path of continual development and learning for the practitioner. When viewed as such, the path of Shiatsu can be seen as a spiritual path of great richness.

A holistic approach

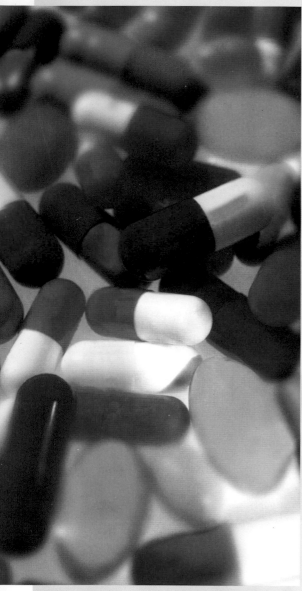

Shiatsu has no negative side effects – unlike painkillers.

When you get a headache, what is your first reaction? Is it to reach for the painkillers and then to carry on as best you can? This reaction typifies a fairly standard way of thinking, in which the symptom is being treated and not the cause of the problem.

Treating the effect, rather than the cause, is normally a temporary measure. If you continually mask symptoms with painkillers, you may be hiding an underlying problem that could have been treated before it became serious. There is also the possibility that the medicines themselves may build up and form toxins within your body.

A qualified Shiatsu practitioner will always try to look beyond the effect and into the cause of a problem. Shiatsu therapists use their treatments to peel away the layers gradually and to treat on a very deep level.

This will happen through the process of allowing Ki to flow better. The flow of Ki, when unrestricted, will help to maintain a healthy body, mind and spirit. A Shiatsu therapist will not use any drugs or medications. This prevents toxins from entering the body during treatment and can additionally be beneficial to the recipient.

In its perfect form, Shiatsu is a method that can help by treating on a variety of different levels to aid healing. This multi-level treatment can then help recipients to heal areas of their lives that can be difficult to affect through the use of conventional Western methods.

In this context, I see the Shiatsu therapist as a person who works with the medical doctors rather than against them. I do not think that one could ever replace the other.

Different Shiatsu styles

When you learn, or experience, Shiatsu, you are reaching into a tree of knowledge whose root is known to go back as far as the seventeenth century. The origins of Shiatsu are in China. Shiatsu was not officially recognised as a healing art in Japan until the mid-1950s, when the Japanese Ministry of Health and Welfare gave it recognition.

Indeed, three hundred years ago, Japanese doctors were required to study a system called 'Anma', which taught them about energy channels and pressure points. However, the Japanese authorities had put so many restrictions upon Anma treatment that a new name for the treatment was given, hence Shiatsu.

As you can imagine, there are many different roots and branches of Shiatsu. In a way, it is similar to music. The history of music is long, and there are many variations, each dependent upon location, time and orientation. Whether you listen to Bach or heavy rock, there is always the link that they are both music, whether they are to your taste or not.

Different ways of practising Shiatsu can be very classical, bearing heavily on Eastern thought, or more Western, taking in such modern sciences as physiology and psychology. You cannot say that one is better than the other, just that they are different.

A Shiatsu therapist need not be limited to one way of working. Frequently, a treatment will involve the use of knowledge or techniques from more than one style. What will matter is that the treatment has fluidity and coherence, not that the therapist has rigidly followed somebody else's ideas.

As discussed, there are many styles of Shiatsu treatment. Three of the more common ones are outlined at right.

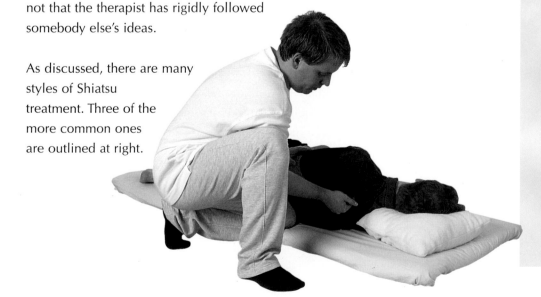

Five-element Shiatsu
This is a common style for the trainee therapist to learn as it incorporates the classical meridian system and the five-element theory. We will study the five-element theory in this book.

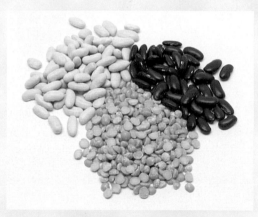

Macrobiotic Shiatsu
The founders of macrobiotic Shiatsu are generally recognised as being George Ohsawa, Michio Kushi and Shizuko Yamamoto. The system uses the classical acupuncture channels and incorporates barefoot Shiatsu. It uses dietary ideas that emphasise natural, unprocessed food and balanced living.

Zen Shiatsu
Shizuto Masunaga developed Zen Shiatsu. It uses an extended meridian system and the Kyo-Jitsu tonification principle. The Kyo-Jitsu tonification principle requires that the therapist can sense the quality of the energy in a Tsubo in order to treat it. Zen Shiatsu emphasises the use of body areas rather than using prescribed points.

Units of measurement in Shiatsu

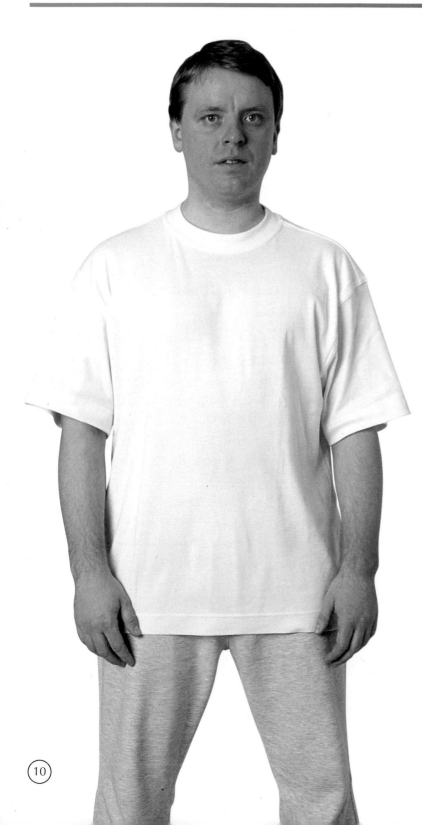

In Shiatsu, you will need to be able to find specific points on the body and will therefore need a system of measurement to help to locate them. After you have become accustomed to following the energy in a meridian, this will become less important, as you will be able to find the points by sensing them. To get to this stage, though, you need to be able to locate the points accurately in order to determine what they feel like from your own experience.

Imagine, for example, that you were trying to find the bladder meridian. On an average-sized woman, the meridian lies approximately 45mm (2in) from the centre of the spine. This is a fine rule of thumb for an average-sized woman, but clearly our 45mm is meaningless for a child or a large man.

A system that can be used for different-sized individuals uses a unit of measurement called the **cun** (pronounced 'sun'). A unit of 1 cun is the same as the width of your thumb at the widest part. There are other definitions (shown opposite) that you can use if you have an oddly shaped thumb. This means that you will always be using a unit that is relative to the person being measured.

The advantage of this system is that you can say that the bladder meridian lies 1.5 cun away from the spine rather than approximately 45mm on a woman, 35mm on a child and 50mm on a man.

Standard examples of cun measurements are as follows.

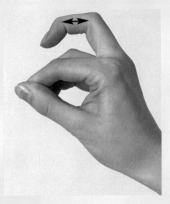

The length of your middle bone on your middle finger = *1 cun.*

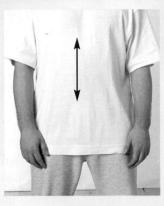

The distance between the navel and the lower sternum = *8 cun.*

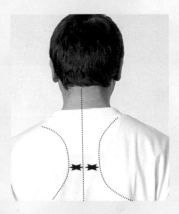

The width of all four fingers = *3 cun.*

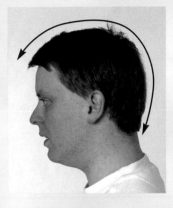

The distance along the head's midline, from the hairline on the forehead to that on the back of the neck = *12 cun.*

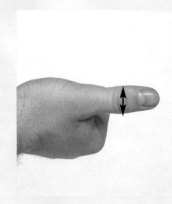

The width of your thumb = *1 cun.*

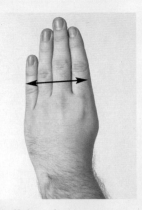

The gap between the scapula and the centre of the spine = *3 cun.*

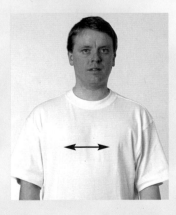

The distance between the nipples = *8 cun.*

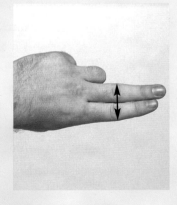

The width of the first two fingers = *1.5 cun.*

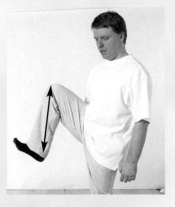

From kneecap to ankle = *16 cun.*

From armpit to top of hip = *12 cun.*

Ki

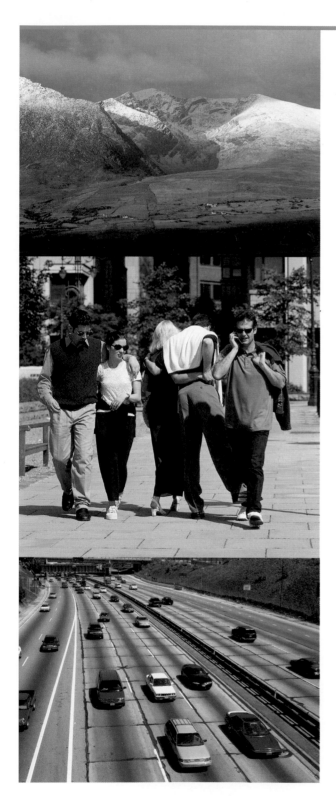

What is Ki? Before answering that question, a warning: the very concept of Ki has, in recent years, become vastly commercial. There are many theories for this, such as the idea that a shift in global consciousness is happening, causing more people to explore such areas.

As a result, many misleading ideas have spread about the subject. For example, healers who can heal with a single touch are as rare as the 'Kung Fu death touch' that was often quoted during the martial-arts craze of the 1970s. Behind the glamorous façade, any healer or martial artist who wants to develop their Ki will have some serious training to do before becoming adept.

The idea of Ki is not limited to Shiatsu. A few other words that mean the same thing are listed below, along with their nation of origin and the person associated with the word where appropriate.

Ki	Japan
Chi	China
Orgone energy	Germany (Wilhelm Reich)
Prana	India
Mana	Polynesia
Vis medicatrix Naturae	Greece (Hippocrates)
Morphogenic fields	England (Rupert Sheldrake)

There are many more names that could also be included in the list. Each represents an individual way of describing what is actually the same thing.

Another word for Ki is **energy.** In the model that we are using from Shiatsu and Chinese medicine, the words 'Ki' and 'energy' are interchangeable. I ask you now to think of the most famous mathematical equation of all time:

$$E = mc^2$$

This states that energy is equal to mass, multiplied by a constant. The constant is the speed of light. This means that when interpreted in this way, mass is equivalent to energy.

This follows the idea that everything is comprised of **Ki**. Trees, people, cars, mountains or even ideas are all made from Ki. Think about this for a while. You are energy. The book that you are reading is also energy.

However, there is a quality that you have, but the book does not: life. The ability to have life comes from a manifestation of Ki, called **Jing**. Jing is therefore the life force that pervades all living things. The book that you are holding has no Jing. When it was a tree, growing in the forest, it did have Jing. When it was felled, ready for the paper mill, the Jing started to leak back into the universe.

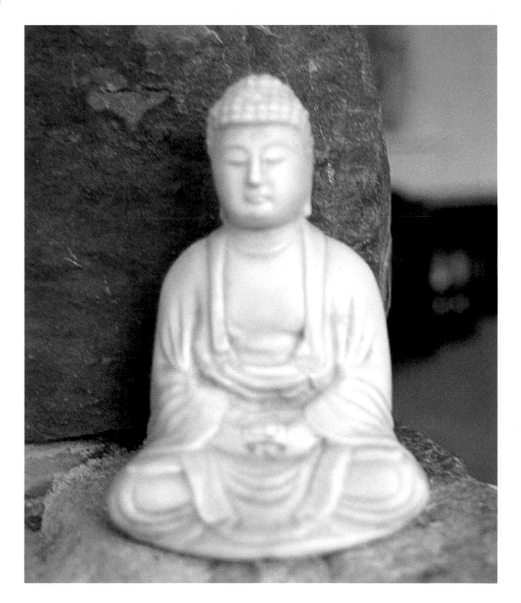

To simplify, when our tree was in the forest, it was alive, but could not understand the fact that it was going to become a book about Shiatsu. It probably did not even know that it was alive. It did not have a consciousness. The manifestation of Ki that allows consciousness to appear is called **Shen**. Traditionally, the only creature that has Shen is a human being. This is because humans were thought to be the only creatures that have the ability of self-reflection.

I prefer to think of different levels of Shen. For example, a dog knows that it is a dog and not a cat, so it must have some degree of self-reflection to know this. Conversely, I have still not seen a dog reading Sartre and trying to reflect on the nature of things!

Yin and Yang

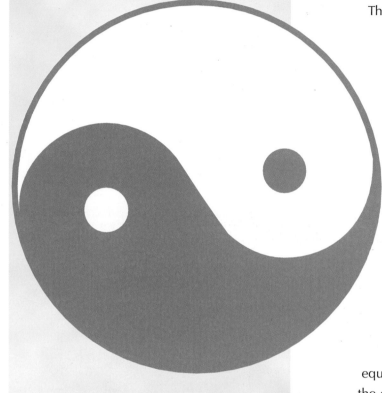

The Taoist idea of creation states that at the beginning of the universe there was nothing. Gradually, the forces of Yin and Yang began to appear as opposites. They joined together in a myriad of different ways to form the 'ten thousand things', or our universe.

This goes back to our definition of Ki. The idea here is that matter and energy are different versions of the same entity. We have gone slightly further, saying that for anything to exist there must be two opposite polarities to the energy, and we have given these the names Yin and Yang.

This may remind you of something that you may have learned about atoms during your schooldays. An atom is made from protons, neutrons and electrons. Protons are positive, electrons are negative and neutrons are neutral. The reason why some particles are neutral is because they carry equal positive and negative charges, each therefore cancelling out the other's charge. This means that the atoms that we are made from consist of two different energies that are oppositely polarised – another way of saying that everything is made up from a combination of Yin and Yang energies.

The parallels between modern physics and Taoism continue further, but this should give you an idea of where Yin and Yang originate.

So what will that mean to us? It is helpful in many ways. The balance between rising and falling, left and right, love and hate, input and output, day and night, asleep and awake, calm and excited and so on are some of the ideas that a therapist will think about and work on. There is also the idea that when Yin becomes extreme it becomes Yang, and vice versa.

The idea of balance is useful to the therapist, and the concept of Yin and Yang can be helpful because it provides a theoretical basis upon which to work. The idea becomes potent when you consider that it is actually the way that the universe works.

What is a meridian?

All humans are filled with a certain quantity of blood. The blood nourishes our internal organs and performs many other functions. Blood is not static, but it is pumped through our systems via a system of veins and arteries. These veins and arteries are the pathways through which your blood can travel to do its work.

A similar idea exists for our energy, which needs its own pathways or channels. These channels are frequently referred to as 'meridians'. The energy meridians are invisible, but qualities of the energy within them can be detected in many ways by the trained Shiatsu therapist.

Meridians do not exist in the sense that a surgeon would see their pathways during an operation. Their presence has, however, been tested by many scientists, who have found evidence that seems to back up the theory that they exist. For example, radioactive isotopes will travel along a meridian pathway when injected into an acupoint. Injections into areas that are not on a meridian pathway do not produce similar results.

Meridians are connected together in Yin and Yang pairs to the organs, similar to the way in which veins and arteries are connected to the heart. The difference here is that not all of the energy comes directly from the heart in the same way that blood does.

Each organ has its own meridian and is paired with another organ to complete the circuit. For example, Yang energy from the stomach makes a circuit with Yin energy from the spleen.

One of the tasks that the Shiatsu therapist will try to perform is to balance the energy flowing within the meridian channels and therefore to help to maintain the health of the organs affected.

This is a somewhat simplified 'first look' at the healing role of the Shiatsu therapist. When you study Shiatsu more deeply, you will find that if you cause a change in one meridian, you will affect all of the others, and that all of the meridians are connected.

What is a Tsubo?

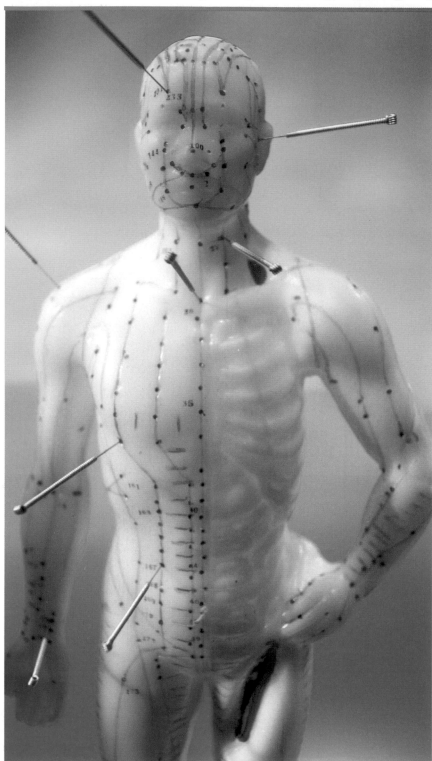

One of the techniques most associated with Shiatsu is the use of acupressure. This means that therapists are pressing the same points with their thumbs that acupuncturists would use to insert their needles in. We know from our discussion about meridians that energy travels in defined paths under the skin. If we are to affect that energy to promote healing, we must find a way of interfacing with the recipient's energy.

One of the ways that we can do this is to use Tsubos. A Tsubo will rise from a meridian to the skin in a vortex pattern. This gives therapists a point at which they can access the meridian energy and work with it as required.

The Japanese character for a Tsubo is a useful image here. It looks similar to a bottle with a long neck and a lid. The neck of the 'bottle' is the path to the meridian through the Tsubo, and the bottle is like the meridian when drawn as a cross section.

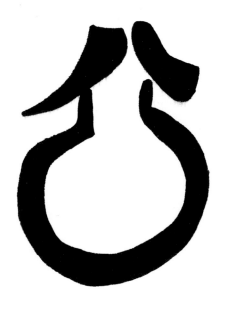

Both acupuncturists and Shiatsu therapists use Tsubos.

Five-element theory

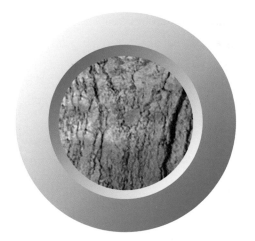

WOOD

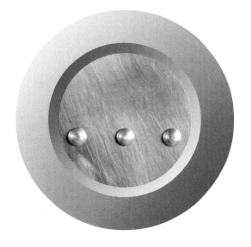

METAL

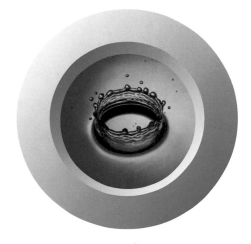

WATER

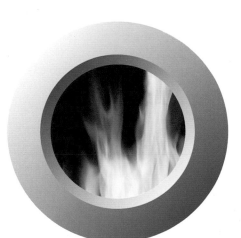

FIRE

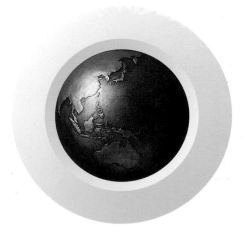

EARTH

Ancient Taoist monks and sages, who observed the phenomenon of the changing seasons, as well as humankind's interaction with the seasons, devised the five-element theory. Through meditation and reflection, they developed a theory that split the year into five. The seasons can be seen on a microcosmic and macrocosmic level. For example, a single day can be divided into the five sections coherently, as can a year or even a lifetime.

The idea of an element needs to be understood in the terms that are intended. The concept of an element here is not as a material object, as in Western science. It is more accurate to think of the elements as movements, or phases, of energy. This is a good approach, as the very suggestion of phases or movements implies that energy is changing from one state to another.

The five elements each have a name: fire, earth, metal, water and wood. Astrologers will note here that some of the Chinese elements have the same names as the elemental signs in astrology. It is true that the concept of the element can be used in a similar way to help to understand psychological and physiological factors. It would be misleading, however, to think that the two are interchangeable. Parallels certainly do exist, but there are also differences.

We now have two powerful tools for understanding one way of describing the universe: we have Yin and Yang and the five elements.

The five elements

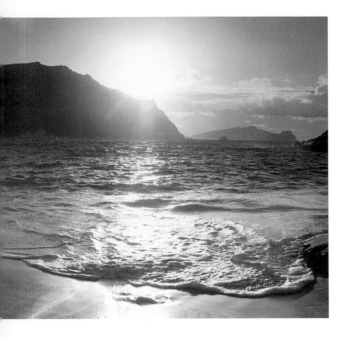

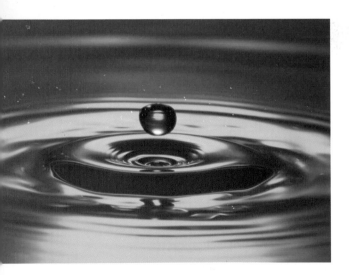

Water is the primal force that shapes our physical, sociological and emotional landscapes.

Each of the five elements or phases of energy has different organs, colours, sounds and concepts attached to them.

In order to understand the use of the five elements and their interaction, we need to develop an idea of the elements and how they work with each other.

Before you read the next section, take five pieces of blank paper and write the name of one of the five elements on each sheet. Now have a brainstorming session and write down as many different connections with the word as you can. At this stage, we are not trying to define the organs within the elements, but if you already have some ideas, put them down.

The connections can be as simple or as lateral as you like. For example, the connection of rivers with the water element is not difficult to make. Then think about the different stages of the river as it rushes off the mountainside, runs through a valley and eventually meanders into the sea.

Then think about language and the phrases that you hear. 'I can feel it in my water' is a phrase that is not uncommon in colloquial speech. This is easy to interpret as being the water element, because the water element is linked with intuition. If you try this experiment and listen for such phrases in your everyday life, you may find it surprising that you already have a good idea of the five elements already.

In the following passages, I have given you some common associations with each element. Following each is a short visualisation exercise to help you to gain a feeling for the concept of the five elements. Remember that your understanding needs to be fairly flexible. In different books, you will see ideas that apparently contradict each other. Try to escape this kind of knowledge and allow the seeds of the ideas inside yourself to germinate and bring you knowledge. In this way, you will rise above any apparent contradictions.

The wood element

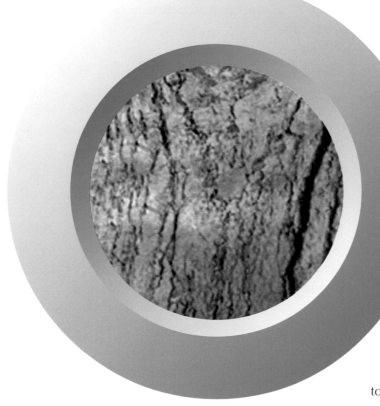

The majesty of a fully mature oak tree gives a
sense that it is the 'ruler' of trees.

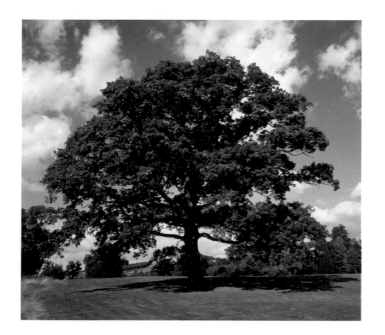

**The energy of the wood element is rapidly expanding and
can build up under pressure.**

Common associations with the wood element

The colour green; infancy and childhood; morning; spring;
new growth; trees; saplings; the planet Jupiter; decision-
making; sight; emotional sensitivity; organising; storage;
distribution; planning; the wind; detoxification;
metamorphosis; distribution of Ki; controlling;
humour; creativity; eyes; jealousy; intelligence; anger;
aspiration; hurrying; independence; kindness.

Wood visualisation exercise

Imagine a sapling as it starts to grow in the spring. The
creative force of its growth can take it from being a
small plant to a huge oak tree. When allowed full
growth, the plant can be an awesome expression of
nature's glory.

Now imagine that something has been placed on the plant to try
to restrict its growth. Without moisture and light it will wither away
and die. If it can gain enough light and heat the plant will either build
up enough energy eventually to push through or else will grow in a
restricted manner.

Now imagine that your ideas are like the plant. With no restrictions,
you can follow your ideas and learn from your attempts at growth. You
may well encounter obstacles, but if your ideas are supported by
enough light and warmth, you will overcome these obstacles and
become fulfilled.

If the obstacles are too much for you and you do not find the support
that you need, then your ideas and energy may turn inwards. This can
cause anger and jealousy to become locked into your mind, in turn
leading to physiological and psychological problems. A healthy release
for your wood energy is therefore vital for your well-being.

The fire element

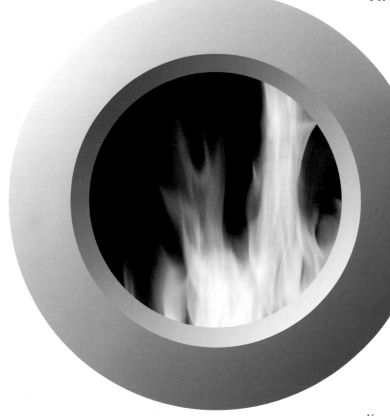

Fire represents warmth, light and joyfulness. It is the extreme of Yang energy and represents energy at its most ethereal.

Common associations with the fire element

The colour red; sunshine; youthful time of life; brightness; can burn out if not sustained and controlled; integration; speech; summer; expansion at its peak; noon; activity at a maximum; growth; meditation; the direction south; the planet Mars.

Fire visualisation exercise

Imagine, or watch, a fire starting. At first the flames struggle to take hold. Gradually, and with an increasing sense of purpose, the flames take a hold and the fire starts to burn properly.

Feel the warmth from the fire as it heats through to your very core. Do not get too close or you will be burned. Yet without the warmth of fire all living things would wither away and die.

Keep the fire sustained. Gradually throw fuel on to the fire. Do not throw it all on at once, otherwise the fire will burn out. Keep the fire within boundaries, otherwise it will either become destructive or simply dissipate to nothing.

Notice the different quality of the fire as it dies away and becomes hot ashes. Notice the changes in your feelings as you watch the fire or see it in your mind's eye.

A burning flame of passion must be sustained or it will die and turn to ashes.

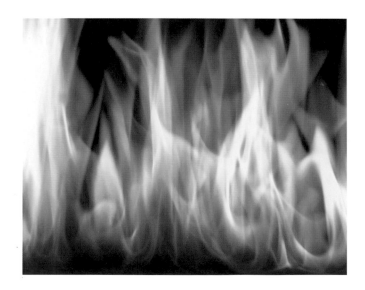

The earth element

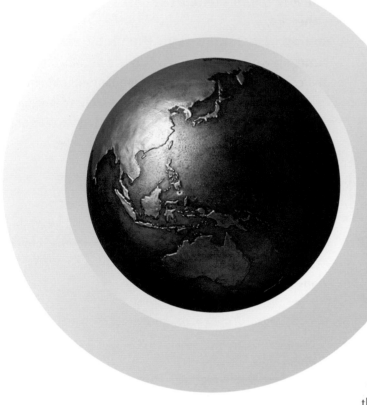

The earth element is represented by the ability to link, nurture and sustain.

Common associations with the earth element

The colour yellow; adulthood; ripening; centre; ground; harvest; late summer; nourishment; equilibrium; gathering; holding together; Mother Earth; taste; stabilising; harmony; transformation; late afternoon; humidity; the planet Saturn; mediation of all other energies; ingestion and digestion of physical and mental food.

Earth visualisation exercise

Imagine or take a walk in the countryside at harvest time. See the fields being tended by farmers and labourers. Observe the calm intent with which they bring the harvest in from the fields. This is not the hectic activity of fire energy. It is more a steady and persevering attitude.

Visit a harvest festival of any religion. An underlying theme to the celebrations will be gratitude to the earth for providing sustenance for the oncoming winter.

Harvest time is the season for earth energy.

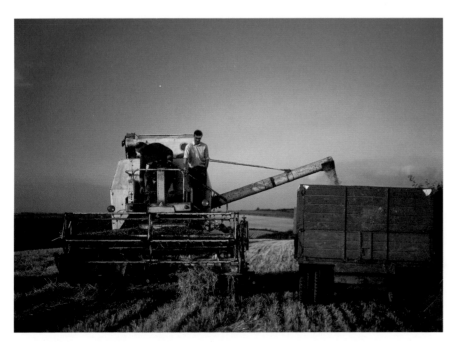

Go out and do some gardening (if you do not have a garden, try helping somebody who does). Think about the earthy quality of working with the soil. Think how different processes in the garden are similar to our physical and mental processes.

After a long journey by automated transport, notice how much more centred you feel when your feet touch the floor. Feel your contact with the earth and try to keep it with you mentally whenever you can.

The metal element

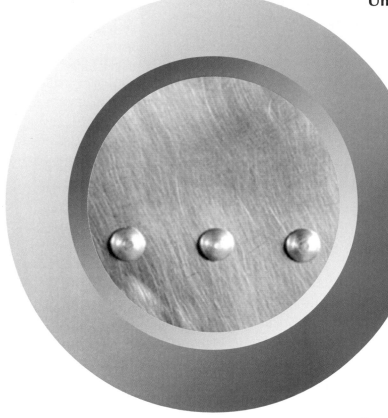

Although the energy of a crystal is very pure, it is 'locked in'.

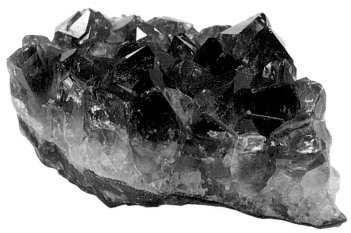

Understanding boundaries, shaping and defining are key qualities of the metal element.

Common associations with the metal element

The colour white, old age; autumn; late evening/night; sharpness; yawning; reduction; elimination; rotting; sense of loss as summer disappears; sense of smell; dryness; the planet Venus; contraction; completion: exchange; energy changing from Yin to Yang.

Metal visualisation exercise

Hold a crystal (quartz or diamond) and cast your mind's eye into it. Imagine how energy is locked into the lattice structure of the crystal. Feel the hardness of the crystal, as well as its defined boundaries with the outside world.

Imagine your sense of isolation if you were like the crystal and all of your energy was 'locked in' so that you could not interact with the outside world.

Remember the end of the year, and the sense of completion that comes with the closing year, with a hint of expectation for the coming year.

Imagine the empty fields waiting for ploughing. Also imagine the farmer calculating whether the harvest was a successful one or not.

The water element

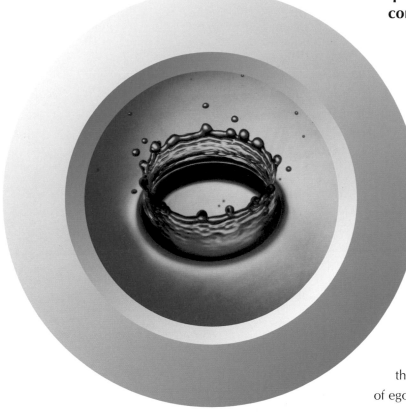

The power of the water element lies in the power to conceive, concentrate and conserve.

Common associations with the water element

The colours black and blue; winter; old age/death; sense of hearing; late night/early morning; the planet Mercury; cold; settling like water at the lowest point; stem; ice; snow; outwardly static, inwardly moving; life in its primal state; intent; the unconscious mind; flowing water; stagnant water; the dormant seed; gentleness; support; fear; spontaneity; purification; cleansing; original Ki; gathering.

Water visualisation exercise

Go for a swim or imagine doing so. As you dive under the water, notice how it becomes more difficult to feel where your body finishes and the water starts. This is a similar loss of boundary that can happen with fire energy. You feel that you become a part of the flow of the water rather than experiencing the more ethereal dissolution of fire. This loss of ego has been utilised by many cultures in rituals like baptism.

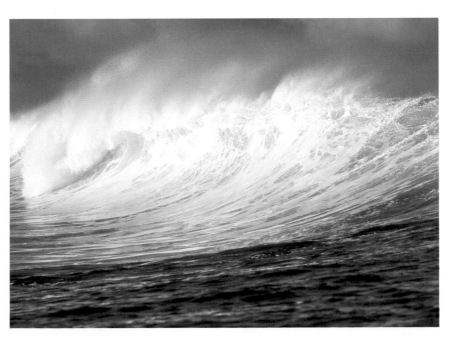

Many poets and artists have used the sea and lakes as a metaphor for the unconscious mind. This could be because these people are usually very imaginative and have an instinctive link with their own water energy. Examine the lives of your favourite poets and you could easily learn about their connection with water energy.

Other ways of gaining an understanding of the different aspects of water energy are to gaze at a moving stream, make love, meditate by a lake or take a bath or shower. The only limit is your imagination, which is in itself another aspect of water energy.

The awesome power of the ocean helps you to visualise water energy.

The movements of the elements – the Ko and Shen cycles

The creation, or Shen, cycle

Many of the concepts of the five elements involve the idea of a sequence. In the five-element theory, one element must feed the other. This element is called the 'mother' of the element that it feeds. For example, fire needs wood for fuel, so wood is the 'mother' of the fire element. This sequence is referred to as the creation cycle or the Shen cycle.

A simple idea for treatment using the five elements is that if an element has become deficient, treat the 'mother' of that element. For example, if a person was weak in the fire element, treating the wood element could make the wood element feed more energy into the fire element. This approach uses the idea that treating one element can help to nurture another.

The Shen cycle of change can be summarised as follows.

• Wood acts as fuel for fire.
• Fire creates ash to become soil (earth).
• Earth contains the ores of metal.
• Minerals (metal) make water nourishing.
• Water feeds the wood.

The Shen cycle is sometimes called the 'mother cycle' because each element nurtures the next.

The controlling, or Ko, cycle

An easy way to think about the controlling cycle is that it is like the children's game 'scissors, paper, stone'. The relationships are as follows.

- Wood covers the earth.
- Earth displaces water.
- Water puts out fire.
- Fire melts metal.
- Metal cuts wood.

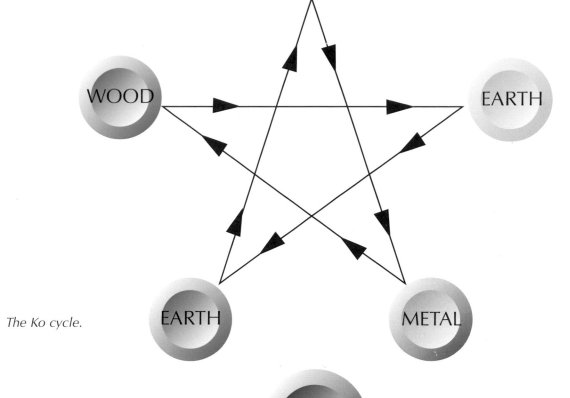

The Ko cycle.

This relationship constrains any one element from overwhelming its weaker partner. Say, for example, that excess wood is in danger of overpowering deficient fire. A possible treatment would be to try to control the wood by treating the metal element. This would help to temper the wood and would therefore hopefully allow the fire to flourish.

When you think about these relationships further, they gradually make more sense. When you have an understanding of the organs and the meridians for the organs, you will understand how treatment of one meridian will affect all of the others.

The controlling cycle shows how the elements control each other.

Basic anatomical terminology

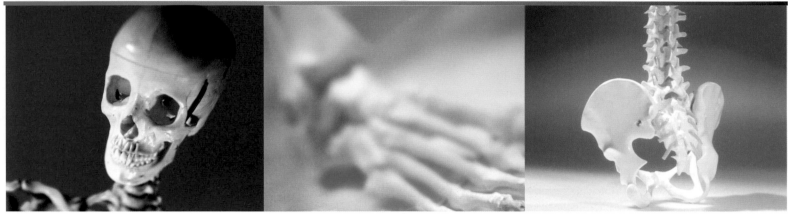

If you decide that you want to study Shiatsu, you will need at least an elementary understanding of basic anatomical terms. It is as well to have at least come across the words used before you start as this will make it less difficult when you need to study anatomy in more depth.

The reason why we need these words is because simple 'left', 'right', 'up' and 'down' become meaningless when trying to describe the human body. For example, if you are trying to describe the location of the lung meridian on your thumb, would it be to the left or the right of the centre line? If the hand has the palm facing downwards, it will be on the right. If the palm is face upwards, it will be on the left. A more simple way would be to say that it is on the radial side of the thumb. This means that it is on the same side of the thumb as the radius bone in the arm.

Common anatomical terms

Radial/ulnar	For arms and hands. Refers to the radius and ulna bones and proximity to either one.
Cranial/superior	Cranial means nearer to the skull. Superior means higher than inferior. These terms refer to the top of the body.
Caudal/inferior	Caudal refers to the tail of an animal. Inferior simply means lower than superior. These terms describe parts that are low in the body.
Anterior/ventral	These two words describe a part as being towards the front of your body.
Posterior/dorsal	The word 'dorsal' is easy to remember: just think about a dorsal fin on a shark. These two words both mean towards the back of the body.
Medial	If you were to draw a line from the top to the bottom of a person, along the centre line to divide left and right, you would have drawn a line down the median plane of the body. Medial means closer to that mid-plane.
Lateral	Lateral is the opposite word to medial. It means that something is further away from the median plane.
Proximal	Proximal is the equivalent of medial, but describes your limbs and not your body. Proximal means that it is close to the mid-plane for that limb.
Distal	In the same way as proximal matches medial, distal matches lateral. It means that a point is further away from the centre plane for the limb.

Your body parts
– a simple explanation of your organs

In Shiatsu, you also need to understand the functions of our body parts and where they are. It is wise to gain an understanding of what your organs do from a traditional Western-science viewpoint before embarking on the process of learning the Chinese ideas.

Try testing yourself. Put your hand on one of your kidneys and think about what it does. Could you remember where it was and what it did? Now try a slightly more difficult test. Where is your gall bladder and what does it do? The fact is that many people have a better idea of what is happening in their favourite soap opera than inside their own body.

Familiarise yourself with the location of your organs using the following diagrams. The descriptions are quite brief, so if you want to learn more there are many excellent books and CD ROMs on the market that will provide you with more details.

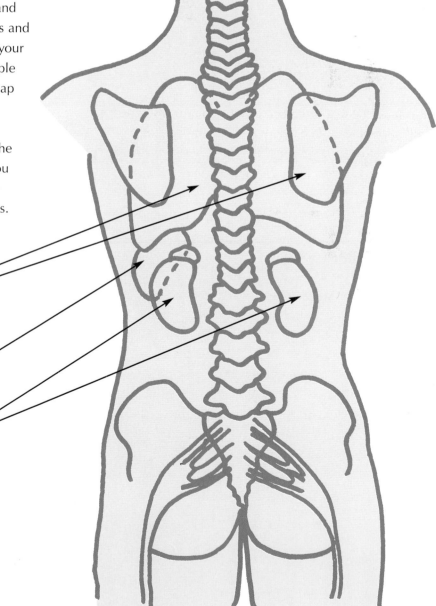

Lungs

Spleen

Kidneys

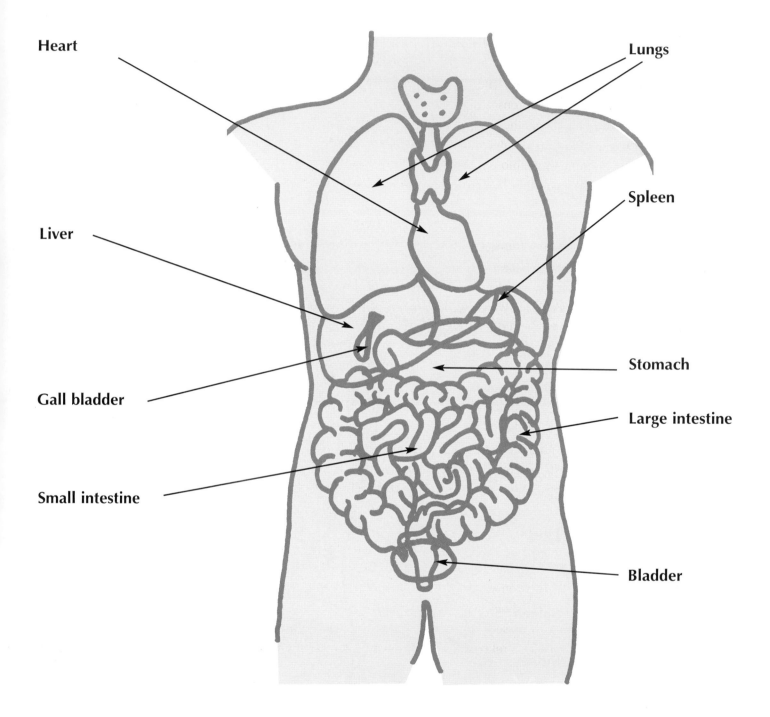

Heart

Lungs

Liver

Spleen

Gall bladder

Stomach

Large intestine

Small intestine

Bladder

The lungs

Your lungs are your breathing organs. They are spongy and elastic and fill up most of your chest cavity. Lungs consist of a mass of tubes called bronchioles. They branch like the twigs of a tree and become finer and finer until they end up as alveoli. The alveoli give the surface area for gaseous exchange into the blood. Movement of the diaphragm draws in air.

The large intestine

The large intestine consists of the colon and the rectum. By the time food reaches the colon, the main products of digestion have been absorbed. The remaining mass is mainly water and unusable materials. The colon absorbs the remaining water, leaving the solid faeces that passes to the rectum and out through the anus.

The kidneys

The basic function of the kidneys is the pressurised filtration of your body fluids. The waste product is then excreted as urine.

Another important function of the kidneys is to help to maintain the delicate balance of water in the blood. They therefore act as regulatory organs, as well as excretory organs.

The bladder

Your bladder is connected to your kidneys via pipes called urethers. The waste product from the kidneys' filtration of blood is passed through the ureters, to be stored temporarily in the bladder. The waste product is urine. Urine is then passed out from the bladder when the lower sphincter muscle is relaxed.

The liver

An important function of the liver is to store sugar in the form of glycogen. It also uses this function to regulate the amount of sugar that is passed into the body, thereby ensuring that it is not all used at once.

The liver has many other functions, including the storage of iron, the formation of fibrinogen and detoxification.

The gall bladder

The gall bladder is positioned on the liver and its function is the storage and excretion of bile. Bile is a green fluid that breaks up fats so that enzymes can digest them.

The heart

Your heart is responsible for pumping blood through your body. Oxygenated blood enters the heart on the left side from the lungs and is then pumped to your head and body through the aorta artery.

On the other side, deoxygenated blood is pumped via the pulmonary artery to your lungs.

The small intestine

Your small intestine is a long tube that varies in diameter due to its contraction. Its two functions are to finish digestion and absorb the products. The first section is called the duodenum and is concerned with digestion and the second section is called the ileum and deals with absorption.

The stomach

Your stomach is a muscular sac with extendable walls. Its primary function is the early stages of digestion. Food passes to the small intestine via a sphincter muscle called the pylorus. Food is broken down in the stomach by gastric juices that are formed by glands in the stomach walls.

The spleen

Your spleen's main function is to act as a filter for the blood and to make antibodies. An enlarged spleen is a sign that doctors look for as an indicator that there may be disease in other parts of the body.

The Shiatsu way of understanding your organs

Where is your mind? We all know that our brains are in our heads, but is that the whole story of the mind? What about love? In the West, we talk about different emotions having connections with the organs in our everyday language, but the mind is usually housed in the brain. In traditional Chinese medicine and many other systems, your mind is not just in your head.

Your brain, in Chinese-medicine terms, is more like the central processing unit of a computer. The computer cannot work without it, but it does not do all of the work. This is the first fundamental difference between traditional Chinese medicine and Western medicine.

The other major difference is the concept of Ki. If our organs have a healthy supply of Ki, then they will be more likely to stay healthy. This will help us to feel better within ourselves, so helping Ki to flow better and thus maintaining good health. If the loop is broken and the Ki becomes weak in an organ, it will adversely affect the state of mind associated with the organ. This can then lead to further weakening and so on. One of our aims in Shiatsu is to learn how to recognise and address this type of problem.

The following is a brief description of how the organs affect our flow of Ki and our state of mind.

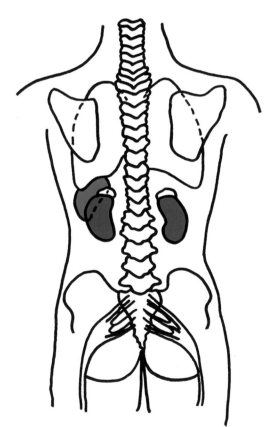

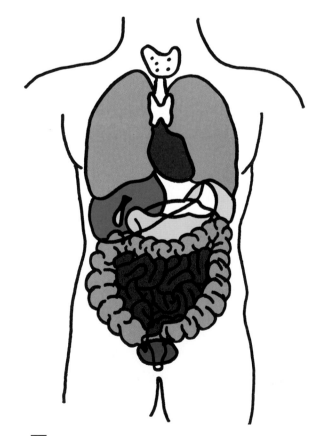

■ Wood = liver, gall bladder   □ Earth = spleen, stomach   ■ Fire = heart, small intestine

■ Metal = lungs, large intestine   ■ Water = bladder, kidneys

Fire element

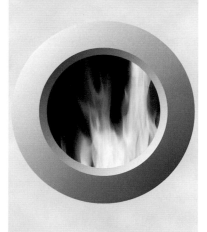

The heart

The heart is the 'king' of the organs. It is the home of the spirit (or Shen), which consists of the positive qualities of all of the organs. Joy, compassion, courage, gentleness and kindness are mixed here to form personality.

We already recognise the heart as the centre of love and kindness. Cruel people are frequently called 'cold hearted' or 'hard hearted', whilst acts of kindness and love can 'warm the heart'. 'Singing from the heart' is another useful phrase in our language, as the heart is also connected with the tongue.

Positive qualities of heart energy are joyfulness, happiness, spirituality, love and respect. Negative traits are cruelty, thoughtlessness, lack of humour, dullness and being hateful.

The small intestine

If the heart is healthy, it can be likened to the sort of monarch who plays an active and vital role in the affairs of state. To avoid being overloaded, the king will need to delegate tasks to a trusted assistant. This is the role of the small intestine.

The small intestine's duty is to filter physical, emotional and spiritual inputs to the heart. In this sense, a weak heart can cause the small intestine to become overloaded with work.

The small intestine is the Yang partner for the Yin energy from the heart.

Other parts of the body associated with the fire element are arteries, the complexion, the tongue, the external ear and the inner corners of the eye. Body fluids associated with the element are blood and perspiration.

Secondary fire

The fire element is unique in that it has a secondary set of meridians associated with it. These are the heart protector, or pericardium, and the triple heater. They differ from the other meridians in the sense that they do not have an organ directly connected with them.

The heart protector or pericardium

The heart protector plays the role of the 'king's messenger'. It passes on the intentions of the heart and gives expression to the emotions. It is therefore connected with our relationships with others. It protects the heart from outside factors, such as heat, and helps to shield the mind from trauma.

Treatment of the heart protector is very useful when helping those with emotional problems. The heart protector is a Yang meridian; its Yin partner is the triple heater.

The triple heater

The triple heater has no equivalent in Western medicine. It controls what are known as the three 'heaters' within our bodies. These are the upper, middle and lower heaters. The positions of the heaters are in the thorax, between the diaphragm and the navel and just below the navel. In our analogy of the heart as the 'king', the triple heater is equivalent to the official who is in charge of the waterways.

The triple heater manages your body's heat and fluid distribution. Imbalances are frequently noted by coldness and an inability to adapt to one's surroundings.

Earth element

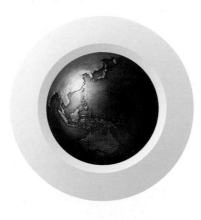

The spleen

The spleen is like a finance minister whose job is to manage the body's storehouses and resources. The spleen supplies the nourishment that we need to sustain ourselves. The main job of the spleen is to transform food into Ki and to transport nutrients to all of our organs.

A strong spleen ensures a good memory and reasoning faculties. Weaknesses can show as a difficulty to define one's ideas and a lack of definition within one's thought processes. Physical weaknesses can show as poor digestion, excessive menstrual bleeding and the over-accumulation of body fluids.

The stomach

The stomach is the Yang partner for the Yin spleen, with which it works in partnership.

The stomach is also a finance minister. This time, the job is to gather the resources rather than store them.

The main job of the stomach is controlling the ingestion of food. This does not just mean the physical food that we eat, but the emotional and mental food that we also need in order to survive.

Normally, the stomach Ki descends to the large intestine to dispose of matter. If the situation is reversed, the result can be nausea or hiccups.

Other body parts ruled by the earth element are the large muscles, lips, mouth and eyelids. Saliva and lymphatic fluid are the fluids ruled by the earth element.

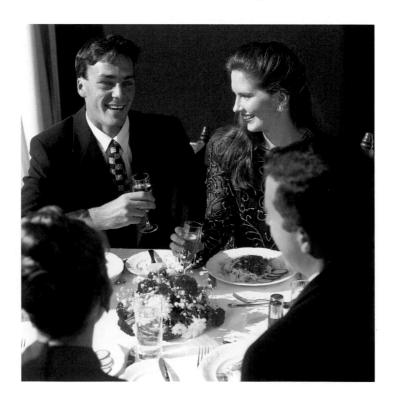

Sustenance and nourishment are key aspects of the earth element.

Metal element

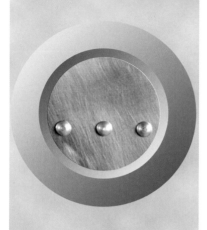

The lungs

The lungs are like the prime minister within our bodies, and can be said to manage foreign affairs and keep domestic order.

Obviously, all aspects of the lungs are connected in some way with the function of respiration. It is through respiration that Ki is dispersed to all parts of the body. If respiration is poor, a reduced amount of oxygenated blood reaches the brain. This can lead to depression or loss of vigour.

It is not surprising, then, that many systems, such as Qigong and Yoga, teach that deep and steady breathing can lead to improved health and a sharper mind.

The large intestine

The large intestine is the Yang partner to our Yin lungs. It is equivalent to the foreign minister whose function is to transform the will of the prime minister into action and preserve the boundaries of the state.

The large intestine receives matter from the small intestine, taking out any usable portions and rejecting the rest beyond the boundary of the body.

Physical symptoms of imbalance can manifest themselves as constipation or diarrhoea. The emotional equivalent is the ease with which you can let go of unwanted feelings and attachments. For example, not letting go of grief can cause a person to feel isolated and hard, like metal.

The metal element also controls your nose, sinuses, bronchi, skin, body hair and mucous secretions.

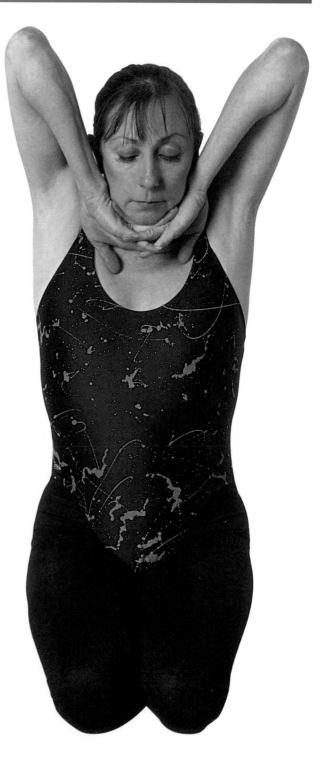

Techniques like Yoga teach that correct breathing is vital for good health.

Water element

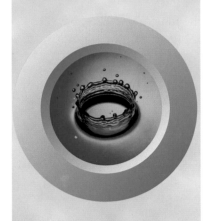

The bladder

The bladder meridian is a Yang meridian coupled with the Yin kidney meridian. Its equivalent role would be a local-government minister whose regions of control are the autonomic nervous system, purification and the pituitary gland.

The bladder meridian's close proximity to the spine correctly suggests that it has a function concerned with supporting the body and with the nervous system travelling through the spinal cord. Imbalances can cause bad posture and headaches.

The bladder meridian can also be used as a diagnostic tool by the advanced Shiatsu practitioner as it contains 'Yu points'. These points can either act as windows into the state of the other meridians or can be used for treatment in their own right.

The kidneys

The kidney meridian represents the supervisor of all of the other organs not controlled by the bladder. It is the 'minister' who conserves natural resources (Ki) for use in times of crisis or transition.

As well as their main function, storing the vital essence, or Ki, the kidneys hold the root of our intellect and creativity. They also harbour genetic information and provide the instinct to procreate and survive.

The essence of the kidneys is that which keeps us alive. If we waste all of our kidney energy, then we will no longer have the impetus that we need to survive and our organs will stop.

The water element also manifests itself in the ovaries, testes, brain, spinal cord, bones, bone marrow, teeth, hair, anus, urethra and inner ear. Its bodily fluids are the sexual secretions and spinal fluid.

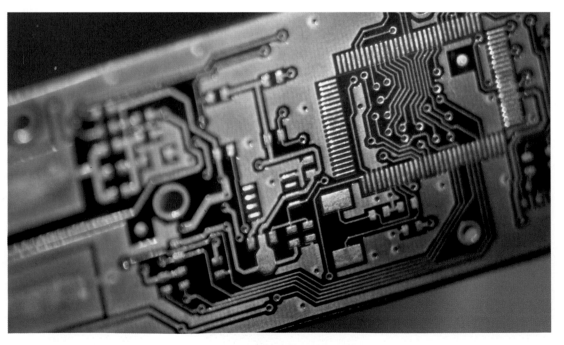

The brain is connected with water like the central processing unit in a computer.

Wood element

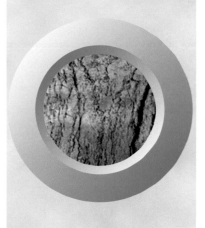

The liver

For this final combination, the liver is our Yin meridian and the gall bladder is our Yang meridian. Planning is the essence of the wood element, so the liver is like a military commander whose job it is to formulate strategies and tactics.

The main function of the liver is the storage of Ki and nutrients. Storage is the Yin function in this case, while distribution is the Yang function. Liver imbalances may show as a greenish skin tone

The gall bladder

The gall bladder is partnered with the liver to ensure the smooth flow of Ki. The role of the gall bladder is similar to that of an assistant to the military commander, who is in charge of distributing information and orders from the commander.

Stiffness in the sides of the body can indicate an imbalance within the gall bladder. This will sometimes be accompanied by a rigidity of mind that makes it difficult to follow a plan through. A weakness in the gall bladder can also result in a lack of vision that makes planning difficult.

Other body parts associated with wood energy are tendons, ligaments, small joint-moving muscles, the eyes and eyebrows, male and female sexual organs and fingernails. The fluids for the wood element are bile and tears.

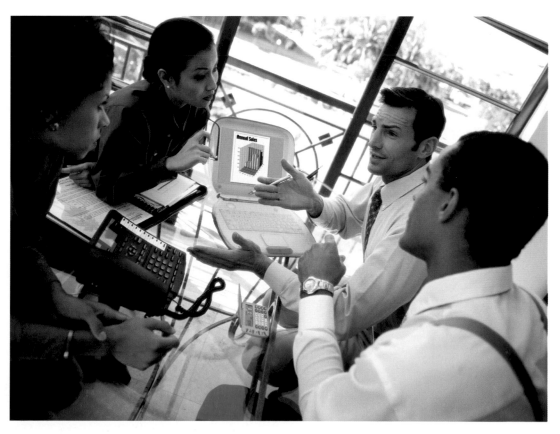

Strategy and planning are key parts of the wood element.

Personalities for the elements

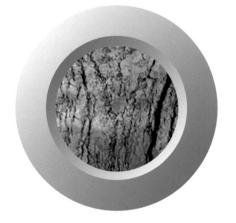

WOOD

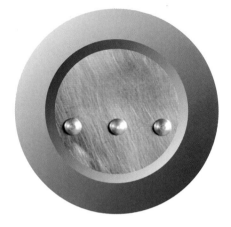

METAL

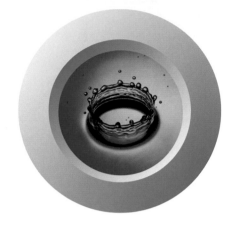

WATER

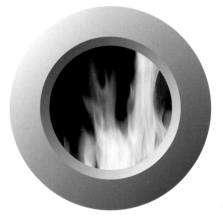

FIRE

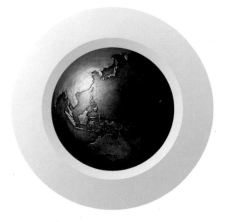

EARTH

Most people will have a dominant element in their personality make-up. We are all combinations of all of the five elements, no matter how well or poorly balanced, but there will normally be a dominant one.

If you can determine a person's dominant element, it can play a useful part in trying to work out what sort of treatment to give. The best person to practise on here is yourself. Take some time to try to work out what your dominant element is. You already have enough data to start trying to work it out. In this section, we will examine a typical personality for each of the elements. In reality, nobody is simple enough to describe in a couple of paragraphs, but we are only using these examples as a learning aid.

When you have attempted to decide your dominant element, try the questions in the next section to see if you can determine your dominant element. When you have found your own dominant element, it is relatively easy to work it out for other people.

A typical water personality

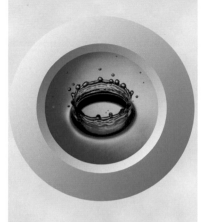

Water personalities are artistic and are generally thinkers rather than doers. They often have a strong frame and a high forehead. Their powers of intellect and imagination are strong and they often have an inner quest to search for the truth behind things. Patience is a virtue with these types, and they are willing to devote long periods of time when inspired and motivated.

When things go wrong for them, they turn in on themselves. Their self-sufficiency becomes extreme and they seem to live inside a cocoon that they cannot reach out from and few can reach into. A bear hibernating in the winter is a symbol for their isolation. They are locked away in the hardness of their emotional cave and nobody dares enter.

At times like this, sleep is the great escape. They will try to stay in bed for as long as possible and, when they finally do rise, it will take them some time to become warmed up and mobile. Their inward-looking nature may also take the form of hypochondria or obsessive hygiene habits.

Just as the winter will finish and turn to spring, so the bear will wake and leave its cave. Given time, these personalities can rekindle their will for life. If they can keep their emotional contact with others, it can help to balance their inward-looking nature. There will always be a need for their sharp minds, as long as they do not smother them with cynicism.

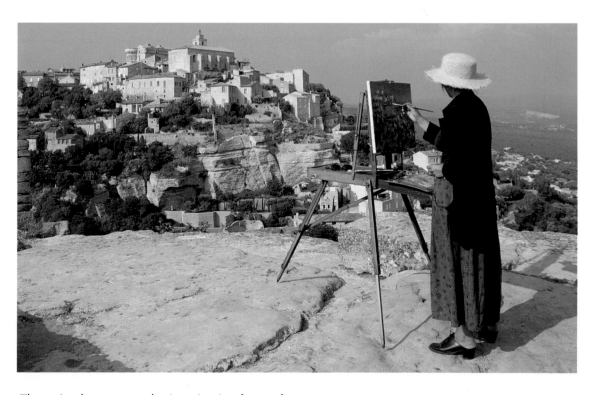

The artist draws upon the imaginative force of water energy.

A typical wood personality

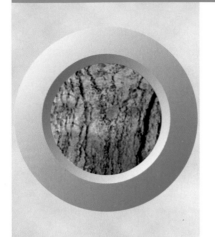

Wood personalities are explorers. Whether it be the more inward type of exploration of the tribal shaman or travelling around the world, they feel happiest when they are travelling in some way. When at their best, they can jump from one task to another at such a speed that many others would be exhausted just watching them. They have no need to work out a situation as within a fraction of a second they can have things organised in their own minds and be ready for the next task.

Inaction is frustrating for this type. Mundane tasks and idle waiting are like poison to them. Unless they can launch themselves at full velocity into the next task they can become frustrated. They frequently eat 'on the run' and use caffeine and alcohol to keep them moving or to slow down.

If they are unrestricted in their tasks, they can be an inspiration to others. Their keen and sharp sense of humour also helps to keep their workmates and friends animated. If they are restricted, or have their plans thwarted, all of the mental energy that allows them to jump so effortlessly from one task to the other becomes blocked, often leading to anger and frustration.

This irritability can cause headaches and depression unless an outlet is found for the mental pressure. The outlet can sometimes be an energetic, and usually competitive, sport or a fierce argument. If this is not enough, there can be residual anger that may make them seem bad-tempered and moody. If they can shift the weight of their frustration, they can very quickly return to their resourceful and ingenious selves.

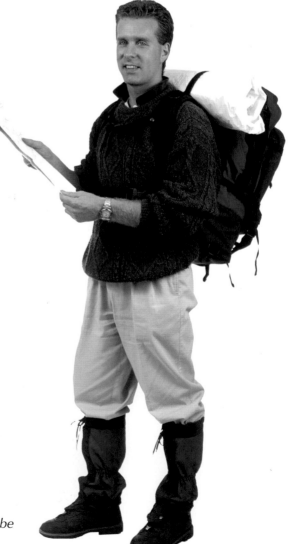

The pioneering spirit will always be present with wood energy.

A typical fire personality

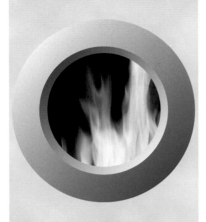

The party never gets started properly until the fiery types arrive. When they do, even the people who do not already know them will take notice. This is not because they are noisy and loud, but because they have a kind of inner radiance that makes people warm to them.

They are good talkers, and before long will have touched everybody with their imaginative humour. A kind of innate sensitivity warns them when not to approach people. When they are at their peak, their whole lives looks like a party to outsiders. They seem to know everybody and everyone loves them for the generous amounts of love that they give.

Those who do not know them well may mistake their openness for shallowness. Those who know them better understand that they have a rich inner life and that they are drawn to many spiritual aspects of life.

Their big problem is that they can sometimes burn up their fuel too quickly. In their need to love and be loved, they can burn their energy down to a minimum. When this happens, they can become discouraged and morose. The time that they allow for rest can be insufficient to replenish them, often making them weak and sluggish. The city that seemed as a playground to them can then look very large and frightening.

To prevent this dissipation of energy, they must learn how to place boundaries on their energy and not to use it all in one brilliant flash.

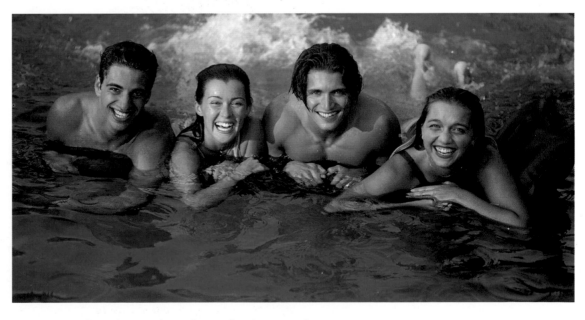

Fire personalities love to have fun with other people.

A typical earth personality

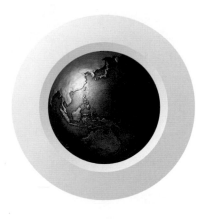

If you are organising a party, it is a good idea to enlist the help of an earth person. They may not be the life and soul of the party, but they will be the bonding agent that brings the group of people together. They are easy people to like. Their winning smiles are enough to bring warmth and to pacify any potential problems. All through life they act as natural peacemakers.

Serenity and harmony are what they strive for. They are very caring people who like to bring these qualities to anyone who needs them. Their many friends trust them, while their ability to help people to reach their core issues can have a nurturing quality.

This can also become their downfall, however. Their desire to please and to help others can sometimes become meddlesome.

Their help may not always be appreciated and may be seen as interfering by some people. This can cause them to question their own values and can make them feel that they are running their lives for the benefit of other people.

If they feel unappreciated and unhappy in this way, their unhappiness can manifest itself as needless worry and self-deprecation. Their unhappiness is frequently buried by comfort-eating, which is then often followed by faddish dieting in compensation.

Earth people can be vital ingredients in creating harmony in our chaotic world, but they must remember to look after their own needs, as well as the needs of others.

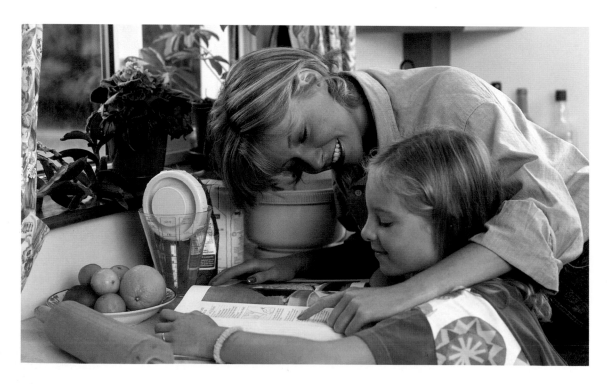

The archetype for earth energy is the mother, on account of her nurturing abilities.

A typical metal personality

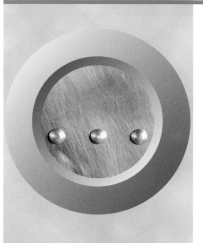

Metal types are generally tidy people. Their houses are always clean and everything has its place. They have naturally good taste and the décor is uncluttered, making their homes feel bigger than they really are. They are not hoarders and do not surround themselves with trinkets and mementoes.

Their working and social lives are similarly neat and tidy. One never encroaches on the other – the boundaries are very well defined. Their specialty is in designing systems. Whether is be systems of working or ways to get around the supermarket with the minimum effort and money, they usually find the best way of working effortlessly.

They are always seeking perfection and use their razor-sharp intellects to cut away dross material to get to the core truth in a situation. Their quest for perfection, however, can be a constant problem.

Nobody can ever be perfect all of the time. When things go too far wrong, they can become rigid and stiff and their lives may seem 'locked up'. There may be little spontaneous action, a more regular, controlled way of life being favoured.

This rigidity can be reflected in their bodily rhythms. Breathing may become restricted, resulting in asthma, and bowel movements are easily affected, too.

Relaxation and breathing exercises are useful, as this will allow them to re-establish better breathing patterns and 'let go' so that they can enjoy life more.

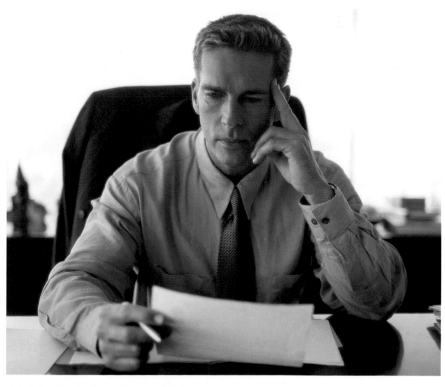

Mr Metal's desk is always tidy!

What is your element?

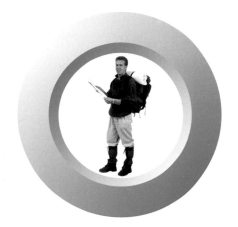

WOOD

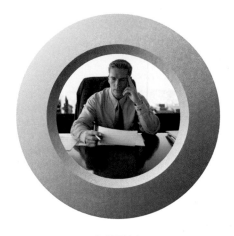

METAL

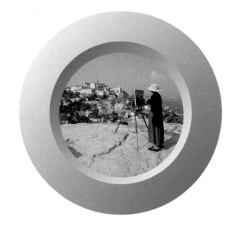

WATER

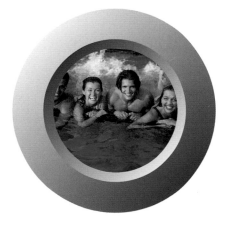

FIRE

The following questions are designed to help you to determine your dominant element. Confusion can arise easily here. The reason is that people often believe that it is their dominant element that needs to be developed. For example, a metal-dominated person may crave the passion that is common to a fire-dominated person, who may enjoy fiery flamenco dancing, for instance. The difference between the two personalities is that while the fire-dominated person will just do the dance and not worry about getting the steps right, the metal-dominated person will have to learn the steps before they can enjoy dancing. Similarly, the metal person must have a pattern to dance to, otherwise it would not be flamenco to them, just jumping around.

It is not designed to be an in-depth style of questionnaire, as this can become unwieldy and can detract from the intuitive aspect of deciding your element. Try to think of other questions that you could include in your own questionnaire.

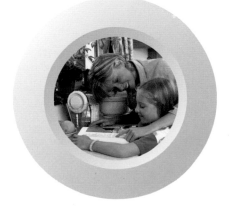

EARTH

Determining your dominant element

I. Do you have a favourite season?
- A. Spring ☐
- B. Summer ☐
- C. Late Summer ☐
- D. Autumn ☐
- E. Winter ☐

II. What is your favourite colour?
- A. Green ☐
- B. Red ☐
- C. Yellow ☐
- D. White ☐
- E. Blue ☐

III. What is your favourite taste?
- A. Sour ☐
- B. Bitter ☐
- C. Sweet ☐
- D. Spicy ☐
- E. Salty ☐

IV. Is your voice
- A. Loud ☐
- B. Laughing ☐
- C. Singing ☐
- D. Weepy ☐
- E. Groaning ☐

V. Which do you prefer?
- A. Competing ☐
- B. Performing ☐
- C. Bonding ☐
- D. Being accurate ☐
- E. Saving ☐

VI. Which is the best for you?
- A. Being aroused ☐
- B. Being in love ☐
- C. Feeling wanted ☐
- D. Knowing that you are right ☐
- E. Feeling safe ☐

VII. Do you
- A. Take risks ☐
- B. Chase stimulation ☐
- C. Prefer comfort ☐
- D. Become judgemental easily ☐
- E. Seek solitude ☐

VIII. Which do you least like?
- A. Loss of control ☐
- B. Boredom ☐
- C. Change ☐
- D. Impurity ☐
- E. Distraction ☐

IX. Which is your favourite role?
- A. Worker ☐
- B. Lover ☐
- C. Parent ☐
- D. Manager ☐
- E. Artist ☐

X. What is your greatest strength?
- A. Your enthusiasm ☐
- B. Your charisma ☐
- C. Your loyalty ☐
- D. Your sense of right and wrong ☐
- E. Your honesty ☐

XI. Which best describes you?
- A. Active ☐
- B. Compassionate ☐
- C. Servile ☐
- D. Masterful ☐
- E. Knowledgeable ☐

XII. Which do you find the most irritating?
- A. Submission ☐
- B. Meanness ☐
- C. Greed ☐
- D. Vagueness ☐
- E. Waste ☐

XIII. Which physical condition do you experience the most frequently?
- A. Headaches ☐
- B. Dehydration ☐
- C. Aching muscles ☐
- D. Bowel disorders (constipation or diarrhoea) ☐
- E. Tiredness ☐

XIV. Which is the worst for you?
- A. Slowness ☐
- B. Inactivity ☐
- C. Being cut off and alone ☐
- D. Chaos ☐
- E. Ignorance ☐

XV. What do you think is your dominant element?
- A. Wood ☐
- B. Fire ☐
- C. Earth ☐
- D. Metal ☐
- E. Water ☐

Now count up your score for each letter. (A) is wood, (B) is fire and so on. Try working out your weakest element by negating each statement. For example, pick your least favourite colour and your worst season. If you do not have an answer for any of the questions, then just leave it.

Your challenges and strengths

If you have followed the ideas and concepts in this book, you will have a reasonable idea of your dominant element. If you are still having difficulty deciding, it is a good idea to try working with somebody who has more experience in Shiatsu. They will most likely be able to give you some good ideas.

For some people, it is easier. It is not uncommon for somebody to be able to identify with their strongest element once they understand what the elements are. If it did not come this easily to you, do not worry: it probably means that your energy is well distributed and that finding your dominant element will therefore be a more subtle process.

When you have worked out your strongest element, what do you do next? You cannot change it because it is a part of your fundamental pattern. Understanding your own strengths and weaknesses can be a useful life tool, however. When you can understand your own life processes in this way, it will be easier to help others using Shiatsu. In this way, Shiatsu is as much about self-discovery as it is about healing.

The following are brief summaries of each of the five elements' strengths and weaknesses.

Fire

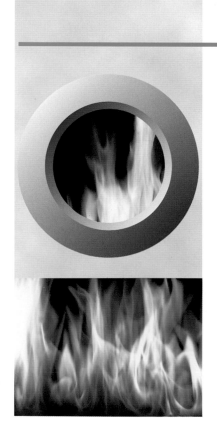

When a fire burns out of control, it will break free of its boundaries. The element that represents boundaries is metal. In the control cycle, fire can dominate the metal element. As the metal element feeds the water element, this means that the water element becomes weakened and unable to control the fire element.

If the heart dominates the lungs in this way, the physical result can be dry skin and coughs. Mentally, the emotions will be in turmoil, and it can be very difficult to rein them in and keep them within manageable boundaries.

Do not let your fire burn out of control.

When a kidney becomes weakened, problems may occur, such as loss of libido and painful urination. This can also cause fire personalities to become easily distracted and doubtful.

Too much fire can also deplete the liver that fuels it, causing stiffness in the joints. The earth element can also be baked like clay and can cause stiffness in the muscles.

As long as the fire type of person avoids dehydration and remembers to try to control their excitement, the fire need not take control and consume everything.

Earth

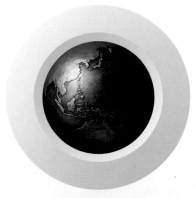

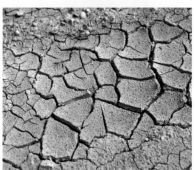

If we look again at the control cycle, we will see that when the earth element becomes overbearing it will invade the water element. This means that the spleen will restrict the processes of the kidneys. Physically, this can cause such problems as water retention. On the emotional side, the earth personality may interfere too often in other peoples' affairs.

The wood element becomes weakened when the water element is unable to support it. This means that the ability to take risks or behave in a spontaneous way becomes flattened, which results in stagnation of the Ki.

The blood pressure can rise because of the extra effort that the heart has to make to drive the vital blood through the stagnation. This can result in the heart becoming enlarged. The ability to draw boundaries can also be lost as the earthy person tries to bring everyone into the family and to nurture them.

A strength of the earth element lies in the power to create links with others and nurture them. However, an earth type should also remember to create and nurture links with their inner selves rather than giving energy to others all the time.

Without the intuitive aspect of water, an earth person can become dull and stagnant.

Metal

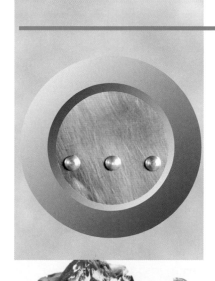

If the lungs become dominant, it can be relatively easy for them to inhibit the heart and the liver. This is because while the metal element displays complete self-control, wood and fire have less control over impulses.

If fire energy becomes locked up by metal energy, a person can become emotionally cold and cut off from others. This can cause heat to become trapped in the system and may lead to constipation and asthma.

Constipation may also occur on an emotional level. This means that emotional problems that should be released are held in. This can cause energy to be locked up in the deepest recesses that may manifest themselves as growths or tumours.

Over-restraint is a problem with metal types. If they can learn to be more flexible and to relax their self-control, the metal person can learn to live with the social connections and passion of the other elements. If, on the other hand, the tendency to lock up emotionally becomes dominant, then their ability to cut through the trivia that accumulates in many people's lives may never be successfully employed.

A metal person may seem emotionally rather cold.

Water

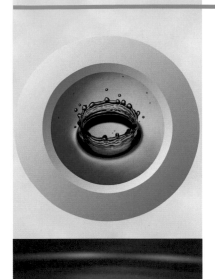

When the kidneys become dominant, they will attack the heart and the spleen. When the heart is attacked, trying to feel love and warmth can be like trying to start a fire with damp wood. This makes the water person withdrawn and can lead to depression.

Too much water mixed with earth makes the earth seem like mud. This will show as weak muscle tone, a pot belly and loose bowel movements. The lungs can also become drained by the excess demands of the kidneys, leading to breathing problems.

Water types can seem very hard and isolated from others. However, their sharp intellect is never under question. If the water type can become more sensitive and soft they will find that their powers of intellect and intuition are invaluable.

Water people should develop their sensitivity to avoid isolation from others.

Wood

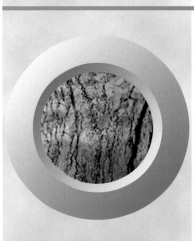

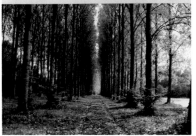

When the liver becomes overbearing, it will restrain the earth Ki and thus upset the digestion. This can also cause a person to live 'in their head' and not be able to ground themselves properly. This can then lead to headaches and migraines.

When the aggressive liver Ki attacks the lungs, it can result in a struggle between expressiveness and restraint. The lungs can also become congealed, leading to phlegm.

The wood type is naturally a hard worker. This may not always be supported by a proper diet, however, and can lead to dietary swings, fatigue and depression.

A wood person needs to learn how to maintain their sense of equilibrium, even when they are rushing from one task to the next. This will give them more balance and continuity with regard to their bodily functions and emotions.

The great power of wood is from expansion and the rapid building-up of pressure. However, this ability to rush forward must be balanced by a sense of knowing when it is right to yield.

Wood people must remain balanced, rooted and centred to reach their full capacity.

Summary table of the five elements

	Wood	Fire	Earth	Metal	Water
Yin organ	Liver	Heart	Spleen	Lungs	Kidneys
Yang organ	Gall bladder	Small intestine	Stomach	Large intestine	Bladder
Colour	Green	Red	Yellow	White	Blue
Time of life	Infancy	Youth	Maturity	Old age	Death
Time of year	Spring	Summer	Late summer	Autumn	Winter
Time of day	Morning	Noon	Afternoon	Evening	Late night
Opening	Eyes	Tongue	Mouth	Nose	Ears
Positive emotion	Kindness	Love	Fairness	Courage	Gentleness
Negative emotion	Anger	Hate	Worry	Depression	Fear
Tissue	Tendons	Blood	Muscles	Skin	Bones
Taste	Sour	Bitter	Sweet	Spicy	Salty
Voice	Shouting	Laughing	Singing	Weepy	Groaning
Capacity	Planning	Spirituality	Opinions	Elimination	Will power
Direction	East	South	Centre	West	North
Smell	Rancid	Burnt	Fragrant	Rotting	Putrid
Power	Expansion	Fusion	Moderation	Contraction	Consolidation
Developed	Initiative	Communication	Harmony	Discrimination	Imagination
Enjoys	Challenge	Intimacy	Community	Organisation	Mystery

The meridians

The following pictures show all of the classical meridians in the human body. You will notice that not all of the points have been listed. This is because a Shiatsu practitioner generally works with whole meridians rather than the specific points that an acupuncturist would use.

Do not be too surprised if you look into another book and find subtle differences regarding the positions of some of the points. This is because there can be variations between one person and another.

The meridian charts are intended to be used rather like road maps. They give you a good idea of where you are going, but ultimately some navigation will be required. Just as you quickly learn a new route if you drive it regularly, you will quickly learn the positions of the meridians and Tsubos and how to feel them. The only secret is to keep practising so that the positions become second nature to you.

The lung meridian

The lung meridian has eleven standard points, five of which are shown here.

Point number	Name	Location	Use
1	Diagnostic point for lungs	1 cun below the lateral end of the collarbone, between the first two ribs	Coughing; regulation of lung Ki, lung diagnostic point
5	Water point	In the muscular cavity on the radial side of the elbow crease	Cold, flu, removing mucus from the chest and pains from the elbow
7	Broken sequence	On the radial side of the forearm, 1.5 cun above the bone in the wrist	Cough, colds, flu, headaches, pains in the wrist; clears the nose
9	Earth point	In the depression on the radial side of the wrist crease	Coughing, breathlessness, weakness in the lungs; clears phlegm
11	Wood point	Near the corner of the thumbnail in the radial direction	Sore throat, nosebleeds, vomiting

The lung meridian

The lung meridian has eleven standard points, five of which are shown here.

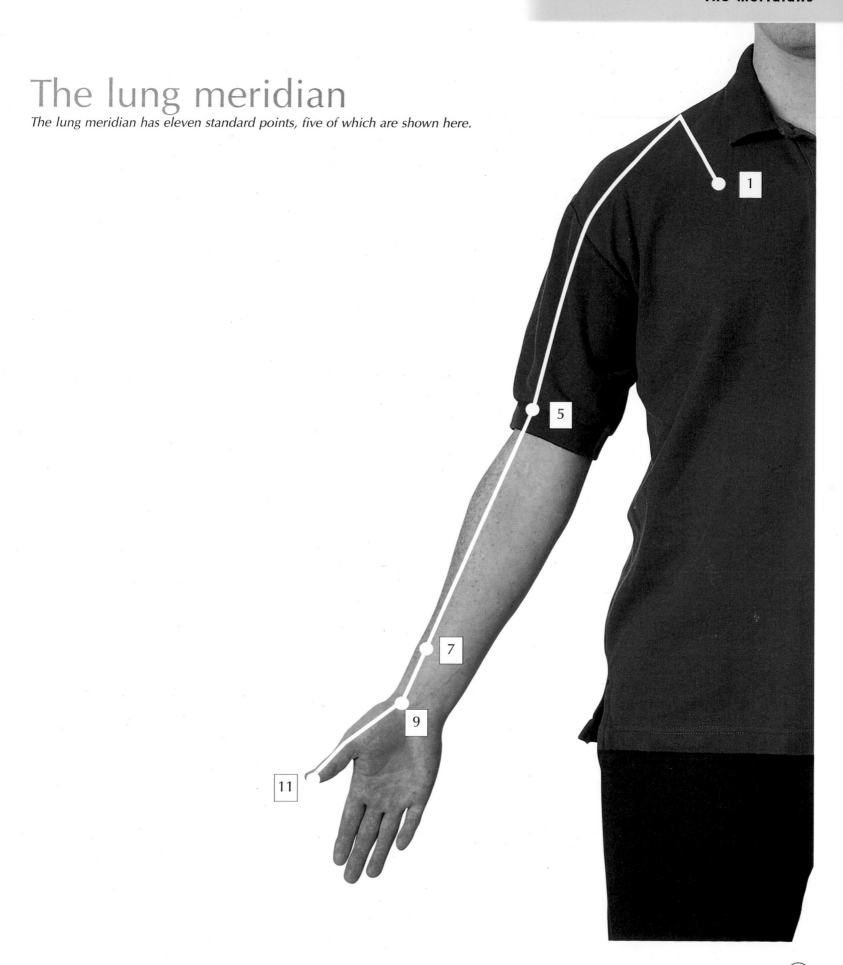

The urinary bladder meridian

This important meridian has diagnostic points for all of the other meridians on it. It has sixty-seven points, fourteen of which are shown here.

Point number	*Name*		*Use*
13	Diagnostic point for lungs	1.5 cun on either side of the 3rd thoracic vertebra	Coughing, weak lungs, lethargy and melancholy
14	Diagnostic point for pericardium	1.5 cun on either side of the 4th thoracic vertebra	Heart problems, palpitations of the heart; calms the mind; dental problems
15	Diagnostic point for heart	1.5 cun on either side of the 5th thoracic vertebra	Insomnia; calms the mind, stimulates blood, enhances concentration and memory
16	Diagnostic point for governing vessel	1.5 cun on either side of the 6th thoracic vertebra	Chest pains
17	Diagnostic point for diaphragm	1.5 cun on either side of the 7th thoracic vertebra	Belching, hiccups, chest pain; nourishes the blood
18	Diagnostic point for liver	1.5 cun on either side of the 9th thoracic vertebra	Gives energy to liver and gall bladder, nourishes the eyes
19	Diagnostic point for gall bladder	1.5 cun on either side of the 10th thoracic vertebra	Nausea, vomiting
20	Diagnostic point for spleen	1.5 cun on either side of the 11th thoracic vertebra	Exhaustion, indigestion, vomiting; strengthens earth Ki
21	Diagnostic point for stomach	1.5 cun on either side of the 12th thoracic vertebra	Indigestion, nausea; strengthens earth Ki
22	Diagnostic point for triple heater	1.5 cun on either side of the 1st lumbar vertebra	Water retention
23	Diagnostic point for kidneys	1.5 cun on either side of the 2nd lumbar vertebra	Back pain, impotence; strengthens water Ki especially in the kidneys
25	Diagnostic point for large intestine	1.5 cun on either side of the 3rd lumbar vertebra	Strengthens the small intestine; cystitis
27	Diagnostic point for small intestine	1.5 cun on either side of centre line of the sacrum	Urinary problems, lower-back pain
67	Metal point	On the outside corner of the little toe	Headache, insomnia, difficult childbirth (breech)

The urinary bladder meridian

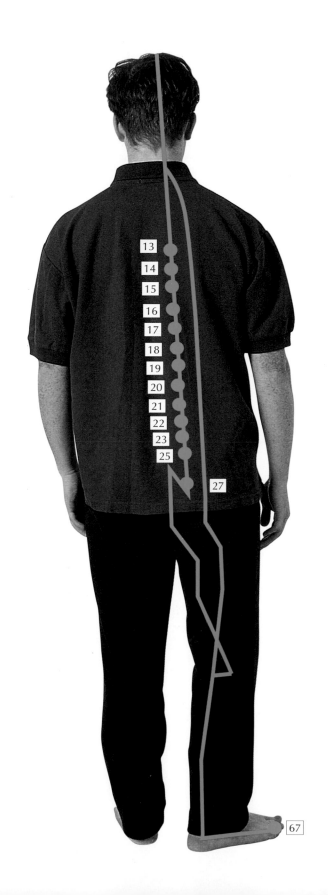

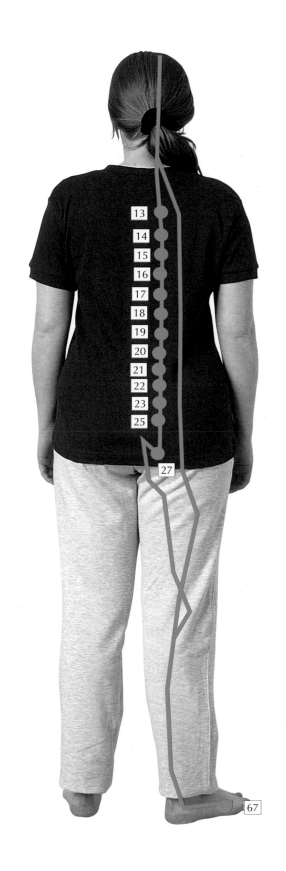

The large-intestine meridian

The large intestine meridian has twenty commonly used points, five of which are shown here.

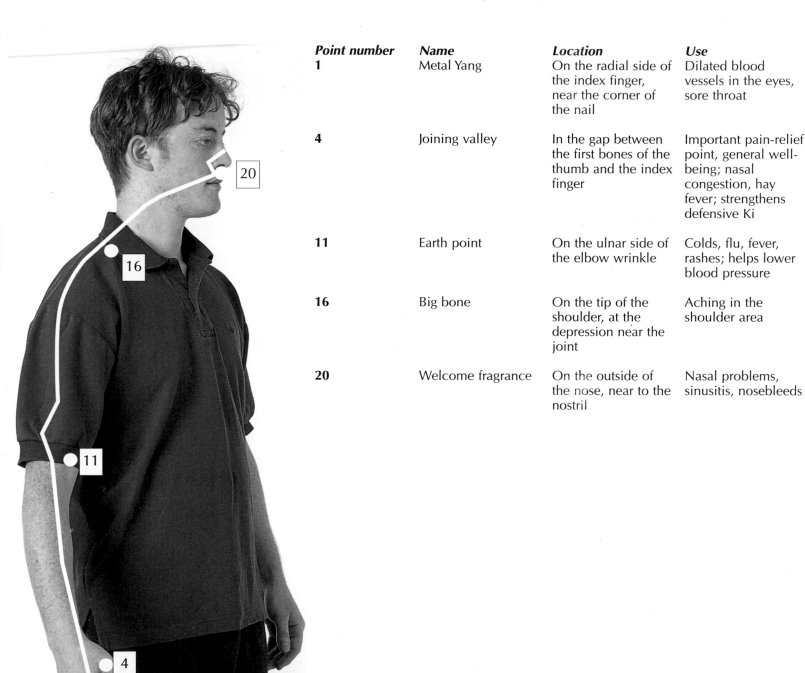

Point number	Name	Location	Use
1	Metal Yang	On the radial side of the index finger, near the corner of the nail	Dilated blood vessels in the eyes, sore throat
4	Joining valley	In the gap between the first bones of the thumb and the index finger	Important pain-relief point, general well-being; nasal congestion, hay fever; strengthens defensive Ki
11	Earth point	On the ulnar side of the elbow wrinkle	Colds, flu, fever, rashes; helps lower blood pressure
16	Big bone	On the tip of the shoulder, at the depression near the joint	Aching in the shoulder area
20	Welcome fragrance	On the outside of the nose, near to the nostril	Nasal problems, sinusitis, nosebleeds

The kidney meridian

This meridian has twenty-seven commonly recognised points, four of which are shown here.

Point number	Name	Location	Use
1	Wood point	On the front half of the sole, along the central line	Headaches in the sides of the head; vitality, general well-being
3	Earth point	In the depression near the Achilles tendon	Any kidney function, sprained foot, impotence
7	Metal point	2 cun above the anklebone, anterior to the Achilles tendon	Water retention; tones the kidneys, reduces excessive sweating
27		At the end of the gap between the first rib and the clavicle	Weak bones; fear release; breathing problems

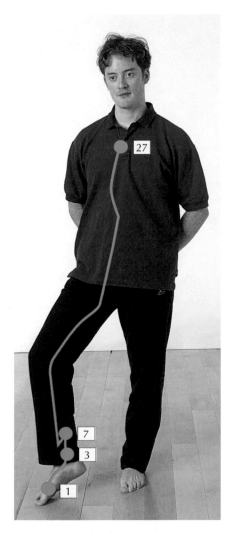
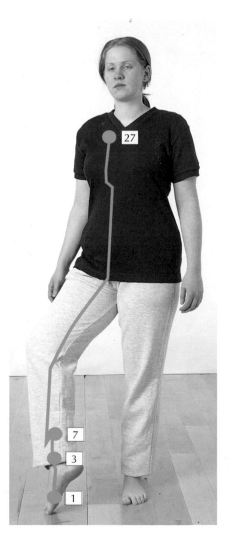

The gall-bladder meridian

This meridian has forty-four points, six of which are shown here.

Point number	Name	Location	Use
1	Pupil crevice	On the outer corner of the eye, lateral to the bone	Brightens the eyes; migraine
12	Whole bone	In the gap between the two posterior neck muscles and below the bony lump	Headache, migraine, fever, toothache
21	Shoulder well	On the shoulder, near the neck on the high point of the muscle	Headache; drops energy to the lower body; stiff neck and shoulders
30	Jumping circle	On the side of the hip	Sciatica, arthritic and rheumatic pains in the legs
40	Mound ruin	In the depression below the anklebone	Gall stones, hesitancy, pains in the neck
44	Foot Yin	On the fourth toe, adjacent to the little toe, at the base corner of the nail	Headache, pains around the eyes

The liver meridian

The liver meridian has fourteen points, six of which are shown here.

Point number	Name	Location	Use
1	Big thick	Lateral side of the big toe, near the base corner of the nail	Menstrual problems
3	Earth point	In the angle between the first and second toe bones on the instep	Cramp, muscular spasms, headache, pains in the feet; calms the mind
4	Metal point	In the gap between the tendons on the medial side of the ankle	Smoothes the flow of Ki; impotence, swelling in lower abdomen
8	Water point	At the medial end of the knee crease	Bladder problems; relaxes the tendons
13	Diagnostic point for spleen	On the end of the 11th (floating) rib	Bowel problems; strengthens the spleen; abdominal swelling
14	Diagnostic point for liver	In line with the nipple, between the 6th and 7th ribs	Nausea

The gall-bladder meridian

This meridian has forty-four points, six of which are shown here.

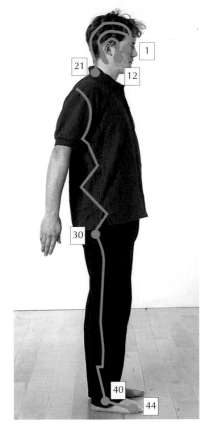

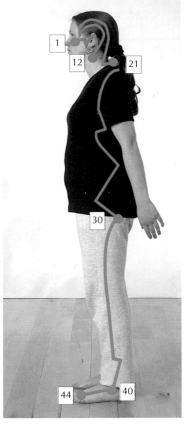

The liver meridian

The liver meridian has fourteen points, six of which are shown here.

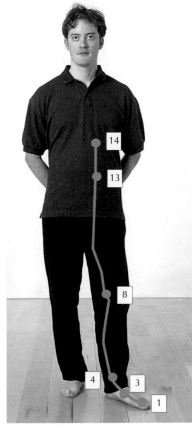

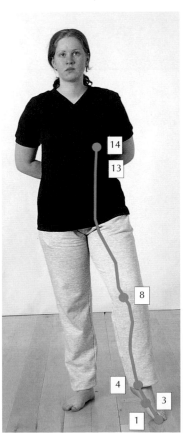

The heart meridian

The heart meridian has nine points, four of which are shown here.

Point number	Name	Location	Use
1	Supreme spring	At the centre of the armpit	Arm immobility; calms the mind
3	Water point	In the depression at the medial end of the inner elbow	Depression, frozen shoulder; calms the mind; insomnia
7	Earth point	On the wrist crease on the ulnar side	Calms the mind, nourishes the blood
9	Wood point	On the inner side of the little finger, at the base of the fingernail	Calms the mind; fainting

The small-intestine meridian

The small-intestine meridian has nineteen points, seven of which are shown here.

Point Number	Name	Location	Use
1	Lesser marsh	Outer edge of the little finger, on the corner of the nail	Headache, sore throat, fever
3	Back stream	On the outer edge of the little-finger knuckle	Headache, fever
8	Small-intestine sea	On the medial side of the elbow joint, in the funny-bone depression	Elbow and neck pain, swollen neck glands
9	Upright shoulder	1 cun above the armpit	Stiff shoulder
10	Humerus point	In the depression above small-intestine point number 9	Stiff shoulder
11	Heavenly attribution	In the centre of the scapula	Stiff shoulder
19	Listening palace	In front of the middle ear	Ear problems, tinnitus

The heart meridian

The heart meridian has nine points, four of which are shown here.

The small-intestine meridian

The small-intestine meridian has nineteen points, seven of which are shown here.

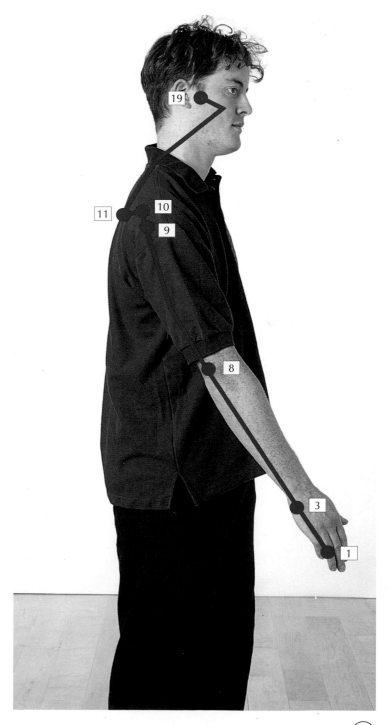

The triple-heater meridian

The triple-heater meridian has twenty-three points, four of which are shown here.

Point number	Name	Location	Use
1	Gate rush	On the lateral side of the ring finger, at the base of the nail	Earache, sore throat, fever
5	Outer gate	On the dorsal surface of the forearm, 2 cun above the wrist crease between the tendons	Fever, tinnitus, ear problems, migraine, sore throat, toothache
10	Heavenly well	In the depression above the elbow	Pains in the arms, swollen lymph glands, sore throat
23	Silk bamboo hole	At the lateral point of the eyebrow	Sore eyes, headache, facial paralysis, pains in the side of the face

The pericardium meridian

The pericardium meridian has nine points, five of which are shown here.

Point number	Name	Location	Use
1	Heavenly pond	1 cun lateral to the nipple in the intercostal space	Tight chest
3	Marsh on bend	In the centre of the elbow cavity	Sunstroke, cramps in the arms; calms the mind
6	Inner gate	On the centre line of the forearm, 2 cun above the wrist crease	Depression and anxiety; calms the mind; period pain, tight chest, premenstrual tension, nausea
8	Lao Gung	In the centre of the palm	Important point for Chi Gung, calms the mind
9	Centre rush	At the tip of the middle finger	Heatstroke; calms the mind

The triple-heater meridian

The triple-heater meridian has twenty-three points, four of which are shown here.

The pericardium meridian

The pericardium meridian has nine points, five of which are shown here.

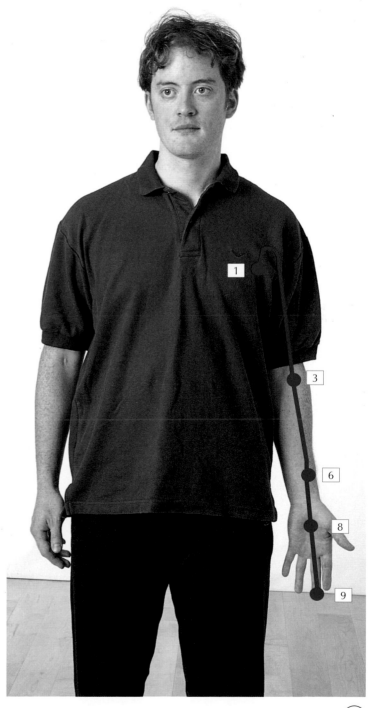

The stomach meridian

The stomach meridian has forty-five points, nine of which are shown here.

Point number	Name	Location	Use
1	Containing tears	Below the pupil, between the eye and the eye socket	Eye problems
3	Big bone	Below the pupil, under the lower edge of the cheekbone	Facial paralysis, nasal problems
17	Breast centre	Centre of the nipple	Not used in Shiatsu except as a reference point
25	Large-intestine diagnostic point	2 cun on either side of the navel	Abdominal pain, constipation; assists the large intestine's function; abdominal swelling caused by retention of food
36	Three-mile foot	3 cun below the kneecap	General point for strengthening stomach and spleen
40	Abundant bulge	Halfway down the leg, lateral to the tibia	Blocked chest, constipation; calms the mind
42	Rushing Yang	Between the bones on the instep	Calms the mind, tones earth Ki
44	Water point	In the depression where the first bones for the second and third toes start	Helps digestion, regulates excessive Ki, flatulence
45	Sick mouth	On the lateral corner of the second toenail	Draw excess energy away from the head; nightmares, headaches

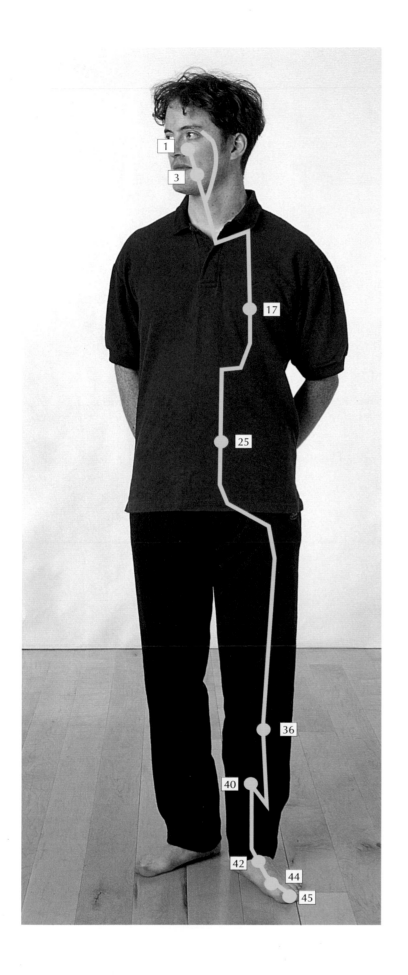
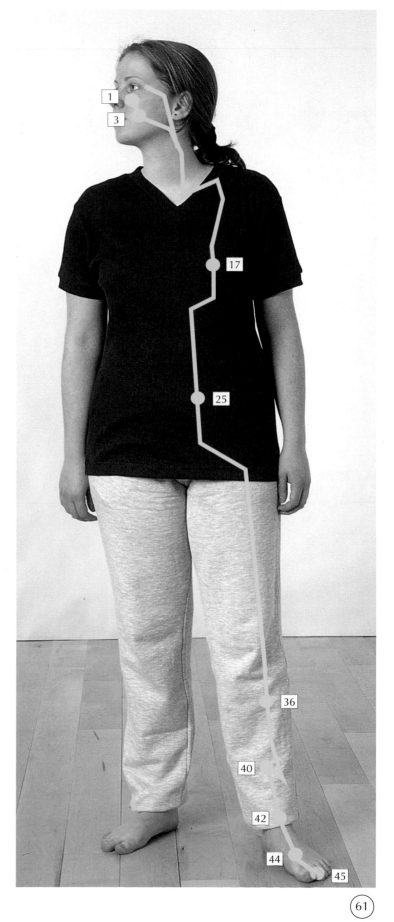

The spleen meridian

The spleen meridian has twenty-one points, six of which are shown here.

Point number	Name	Location	Use
1	Hidden white	On the medial base corner of the big toenail	Menstrual problems; stops any type of bleeding
3	Earth point	In the depression on the medial side of the big toe, behind the joint	Exhaustion, phlegm in the lungs, bowel problems (constipation or diarrhoea), tonifies spleen
6	Yin meeting (the kidney and liver meridians pass through this point)	3 cun above the anklebone	General well being point, gynaecological complaints; tones the spleen
9	Water point	On the medial (inner) side of the leg, on the top of the tibia	Knee pains; benefits the bladder; cystitis
10	Sea of blood	2 cun above the kneecap in the muscle bulge	Skin problems, menstrual problems
21	Control	Below the armpit, in the sixth intercostal space	Benefits diabetics; muscular pain

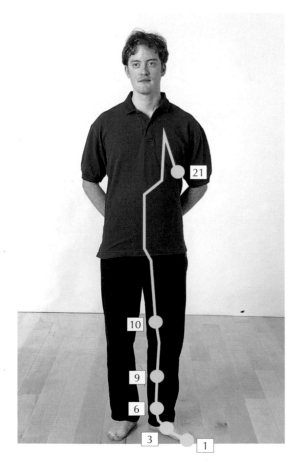

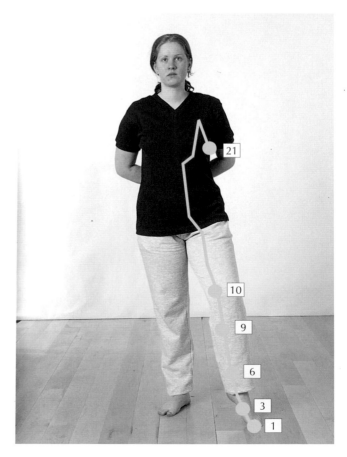

The governing-vessel meridian

The governing-vessel meridian has twenty-eight points, five of which are shown here.

Point number	Name	Location	Use
1	Chang Chiang	Below the sacrum	Helps provide mental balance; piles
4	Ming Men (gate of Life)	Between lumbar vertebrae 2 and 3	Sexual problems; balances the kidneys
6	Chi Chung	Between the 11th and 12th thoracic vertebrae	Gives energy to the heart; hyperactivity
14	Big vertebra	Between the 6th and 7th cervical vertebrae	Stimulates the brain
20	Thousand meetings	On the highest point of the head	Headache, piles

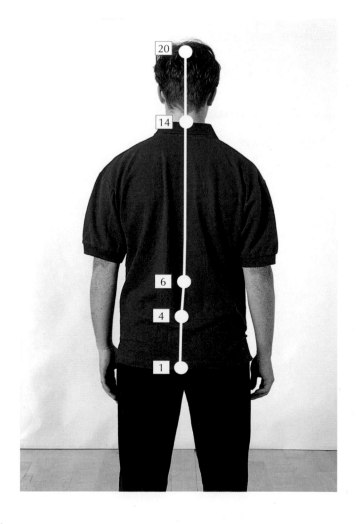

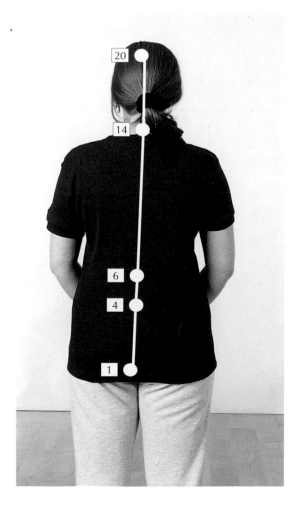

The conception-vessel meridian

The conception-vessel meridian has twenty-four points, six of which are shown here.

Point number	Name	Location	Use
3	Diagnostic point for the bladder	4 cun below the navel	Menstrual problems; benefits the bladder; cystitis, urinary retention
4	TanTien	3 cun below the navel	Menstrual problems; pulls Ki downwards and regulates the mind; back pain; strengthens the kidneys and original Ki
14	Diagnostic point for the heart	6 cun above the navel	Calms the mind; nervous indigestion
17	Diagnostic point for the pericardium	In the middle of the sternum, between the nipples	Coughing, tight chest; moves Ki in the chest
22	Heaven projection	In the dip just above the breastplate	Coughing and lung problems
24	Saliva-receiver	Below the lower lip	Toothache

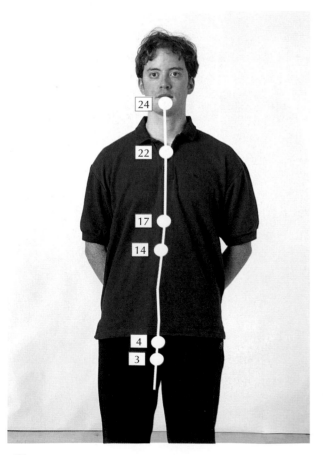

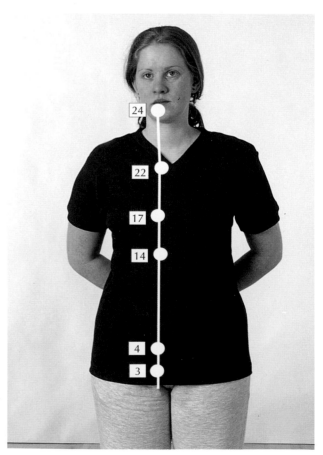

Diagnosis in Shiatsu

In Taoist theory, we do not need to do all of our thinking with the brain in our heads. We also have a second brain, or Hara (a Japanese term), located in our lower abdomen that houses our awareness. This is something that we are already familiar with – we all know what a 'gut reaction' is.

Meditation practices, such as the following, can teach us how to use our lower brain so that we are not relying on the upper brain all of the time. The advantage of this is that while the internal dialogue of our upper brain can be very difficult to switch off, the Hara is not affected.

When using diagnosis in Shiatsu, life becomes much easier if we can use the Hara instead of the upper brain. If you have not developed your Hara, it will be difficult to try to feel your own, or another person's, energy because you have too much happening in your upper brain to make a decision. It will be like trying to pick out one voice in a crowd when all of the other voices are shouting louder than the voice that you want to hear.

This is why an experienced healer will usually make a decision very quickly as to what treatment they are going to perform. There needs to be a process happening and not simply a vague guess. The path of the treatment may even change. If you are in tune with your Hara, you will sense this and be able to follow the flow of the treatment.

This is the same as an expert martial artist who can seemingly predict a movement before an opponent makes it.

There are many methods of diagnosis employed in Shiatsu, and there are several books on the subject of diagnosis alone. Most healers in Shiatsu will know several methods that they can use to back each other up. Some of the techniques of diagnosis are briefly outlined here.

Questioning

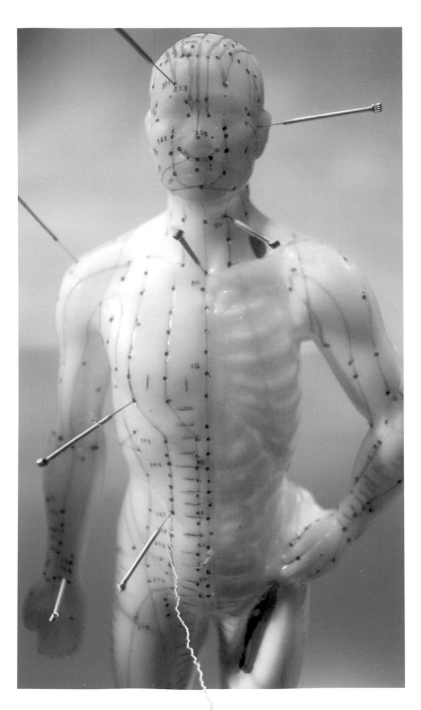

A Shiatsu healer normally employs questioning during a first session. A questionnaire is usually designed by the healer and can then be used as a start for the treatment notes of the recipient. It has the advantage that it gives the recipient a good opportunity to tell the healer what they are seeking with their treatments. The big disadvantage is that the recipient may deliberately avoid issues that are causing problems.

Here are some typical questions that may be asked.

Why is Shiatsu being requested?

What is the current state of health?

Are there any known health factors?

Are medications or drugs being used?

Are there any illnesses or injuries in the client's history?

Any operations?

What is the diet like?

What is the favourite and least favourite taste?

  Salty

  Sweet

  Sour

  Bitter

  Spicy

  None

What is the alcohol intake?

Does the client smoke?

Does the client do any sort of exercise or meditation?

It is not difficult to design your own questionnaire. It is good practice to try making up your own. This will allow you to decide the relevant information that you will need to make a treatment. If you need inspiration, refer to the section describing the attributes of a typical personality for each of the elements.

Listening and smelling diagnosis

When you ask the recipient questions about themselves, it is common for the answers to be misleading. For example, a person with an alcohol or drugs problem will sometimes avoid the issue completely until they have admitted to themselves that they have a problem. In general, if a person has a weakness in a part of their energy, they will try not to talk about it.

This would make thing rather difficult if you were relying on a questionnaire, so other diagnostic tools can be employed. Simple diagnostic tools are listening and smelling.

Diagnosis by listening

In listening diagnosis, you are not particularly interested in what words are being said as much as in how they are being said. The method is to try to determine whether there is an underlying sound to the voice. This is then categorised into one of the five elements and gives an indicator to an element that needs some work.

Learning how to pick this information out of a conversation is similar to a musician learning how to determine pitch. For some it will come easily, but it will be more difficult for others. Do not worry if you have no musical skills as you are looking for trends and not trying to identify individual notes. A word of caution here: it is easy to become engrossed in listening for the underlying trend and miss the words, which can make you look like you are not listening at all.

Basic sounds to listen for are as follows.

The kidneys produce a deep voice. If the voice tends towards groaning, it may reveal kidney weakness.
The liver gives authority to a voice. When weak, it will make the voice sound clipped or angry.

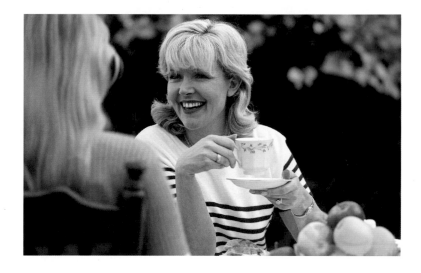

Listen to the tones and rhythm, as well as the content, of the speech.

The heart rules the tongue. This will enable good expression and articulation. Stuttering, or being 'tongue-tied', may reveal a weakness. If the voice has a laughing quality, it may mean excess energy in the heart area.
The spleen gives a musical, singing quality to a voice. If this becomes overriding, a weakness may be indicated.
The lungs give strength to a voice. A voice that is weak or weepy may indicate a metal deficiency.

Diagnosis by smell

Smelling diagnosis is usually more difficult than listening because the therapist needs to sense the person's underlying smell and not that of sweat or perfume, although these can provide pointers.

A stagnant smell can indicate kidney weakness; a sour smell may indicate liver weakness; a slightly scorched smell can indicate heart weakness; a sweet smell can indicate weakness in the spleen; and a musty smell can indicate lung weakness.

Diagnosis by looking

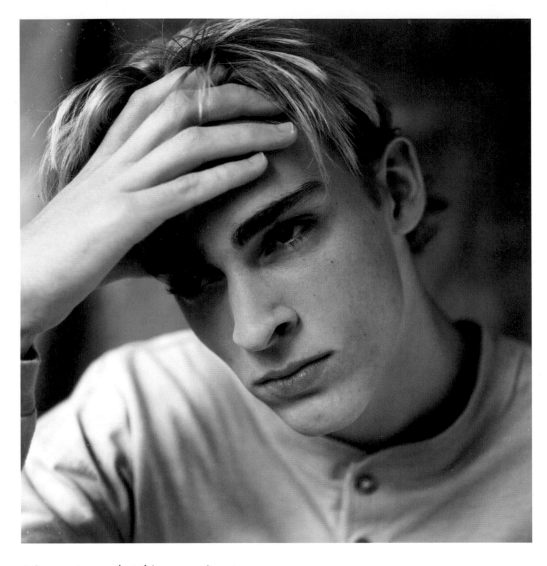

It is easy to see that this person is not relaxed. Other subtleties can be seen when you have studied them. What can you see?

When you look at a person, you will get an impression about them. We instinctively know when a person is angry or upset and can adjust the way that we interact with them to suit their mood.

In Shiatsu, this has become a science. From looking at such things as body posture, body dynamics, distribution of body strength, colour and facial characteristics, to name but a few, we can make conclusions.

Facial diagnosis is a common tool. The general colour may have a tinge to it, indicating an imbalance in one of the elements. For example, we all know that a red face can indicate high blood pressure or heart problems and therefore the fire element. A green tinge can indicate a 'liverish' feeling and point to the wood element.

Facial-area diagnosis is also a part of this toolkit. For example, a deeply furrowed area between the eyebrows may indicate liver Ki stagnation. In the old, classical-era statues, you will see somebody who is trying to show their intellect holding this area, as if deep in thought. As mental activity is linked to the wood element, we can see a connection. Also, if you observe a person with a hangover, this part of their forehead can look puffy, indicating that the liver is having trouble trying to remove toxins.

Diagnosis by touch

Touching diagnosis can be as simple as just feeling the quality of the muscle tone to give an impression of the state of health. In Shiatsu, there are methods that employ your sensitivity to the recipient's Ki. For example, in the meridian locators, there are various points that are labelled as diagnostic points for an element or organ. An experienced healer will be able to sense the energy level at these points and make conclusions.

Another method is Hara diagnosis. There are two common procedures here. One is to use the Hara as a complete map of the organs, as is done in Zen Shiatsu. The advantage of this is that it is very specific and gives an accurate diagnosis very

quickly. The disadvantage is that you need to be quite skilled in order to do it.

A simpler, but less specific, form of this diagnosis comes from the five-element system. In this, we divide the Hara into five areas and sense the weakest and the strongest areas. This is not as difficult as it sounds. You simply touch each of the areas illustrated and make a mental note of what they feel like. If you can switch off, or at least quieten, your upper brain, you will sense that each area feels subtly different. This will tell you which element is weak and which element is strong, thus giving you more information on which to base your treatment.

EARTH *WATER*

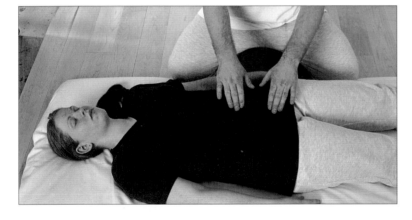

WOOD *EARTH*

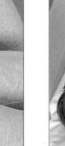

FIRE *EARTH*

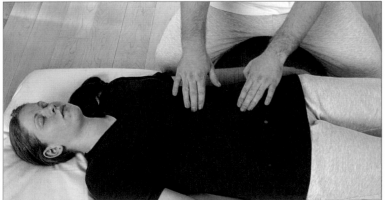

EARTH *METAL*

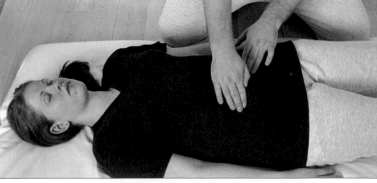

Intent for Shiatsu

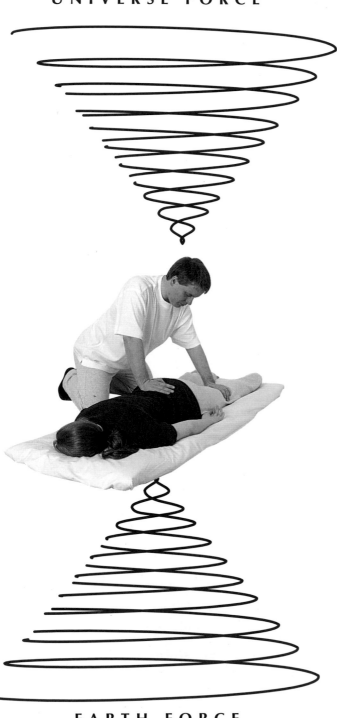

UNIVERSE FORCE

EARTH FORCE

When you practise Shiatsu, one of the things that you are trying to do for the recipient is to restore, or maintain, their healthy internal balance. This will be impossible if you are not 'in the moment'. For example, you may have decided that you need to work with a meridian. You may be one-quarter of the way through that meridian when doubt creeps into your mind. You may start thinking, 'I can't remember where all of the points are' or 'I don't know if I am helping'.

If this happens, it can be like opening a mental floodgate: mental chatter can overwhelm your mind and Shiatsu becomes an impossibility. There is a way out of it if this occurs. Just stop what you are doing and take a few deep breaths into your Hara. This will calm your mind and let you do the job that you have set out to do.

When you practise Shiatsu, you should feel connected – not just with the person whom you are working on, but with the universe. A good visualisation for this is to imagine that there is an energetic opening at the crown of your head through which you connect with the rest of the universe. This is an invaluable technique because it prevents you from draining your own energy by letting the energy of the universe travel through you.

You should also feel grounded when you practise. This means that you should feel the force of the earth under you as you work. Remember to keep your centre of gravity low, and the feeling will be increased. This is why many therapists work in the Seiza, or kneeling, position whenever possible.

If you are grounded, the client will feel that you have a good connection with them.

Preparation for treatment

Before you give a Shiatsu treatment, there are certain preliminary techniques that it is useful to learn and practise as these will relax and prepare your body, as well as making sure that your mind and energy are in tune for the treatment ahead.

If you were simply to begin a treatment without any preparation at all you would not be able to work with the recipient's energy effeciently, so some kind of warm-up – both for body and the spirit – is essential.

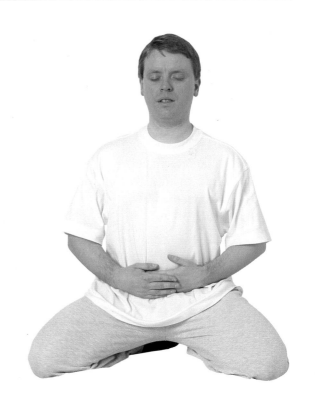

Warm-up exercises

If you have a Shiatsu treatment, you will normally be lying on a futon mattress on the floor. Imagine that you are ready to receive the treatment, but your therapist takes five minutes to kneel down and is obviously uncomfortable giving the treatment. Most people would, quite correctly, think, 'How can he/she give me a good treatment if they are stiff themselves?'

A Shiatsu therapist needs to keep supple and loose in order to work around the recipient fluidly. Otherwise you will be in danger of doing yourself damage by trying to help others.

There are a huge number of warm-up and loosening-up exercises that are practised by different people. The following is a selection that will help you to keep your body in condition.

Neck rotation

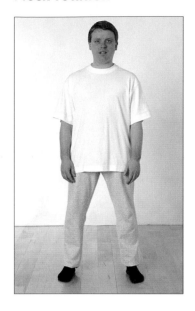
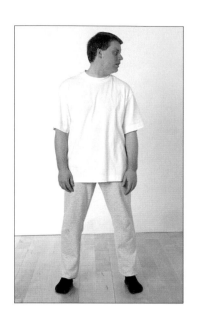
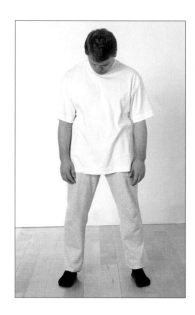
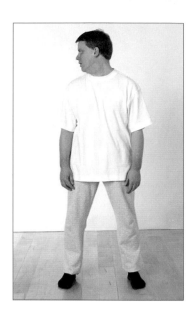

1. Start by standing firmly, with your feet approximately a shoulder-width apart. Lift through the crown of your head, but do not strain. Look forwards.

2. Imagine that you are drawing a circle with your eyes. Make the circle increase in size by increasing the size of the rotation.

3. Try to make the circle as big as you can without hurting yourself.

4. When you have loosened in one direction, come back to the centre and reverse the direction.

Shoulder rotation

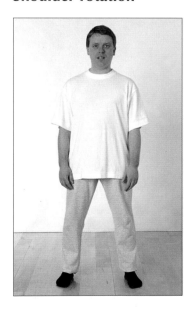
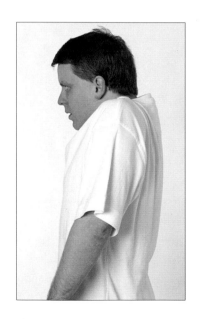
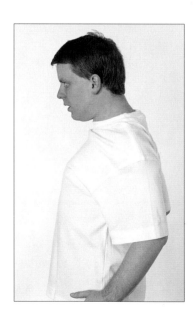
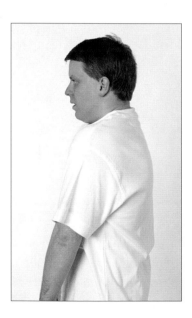

1. Start by standing firmly, with your feet approximately a shoulder-width apart. Lift through the crown of your head, but do not strain. Look forwards.

2. On your inward breath, raise your shoulders.

3. On your outward breath, lower your shoulders.

4 Move your shoulders in a circular fashion and control the movement so that it co-ordinates with your breathing.

Windmills

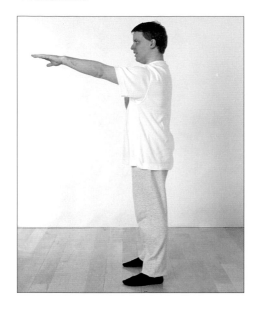 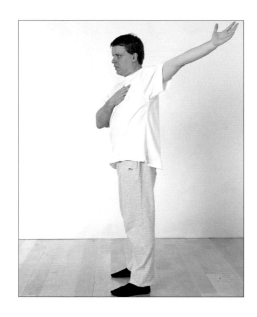 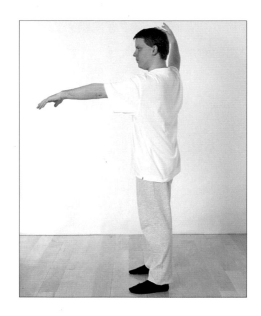

1. Start by throwing one of your arms over your shoulder in a circular fashion.

2. Rotate the other arm in the other direction.

3. You can use the combinations of rotating both arms in the same direction or spinning your arms in different directions. If you find the exercise difficult at first, stop thinking about it and it will come easily.

Waist rotation

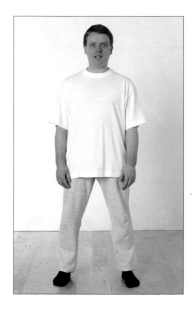 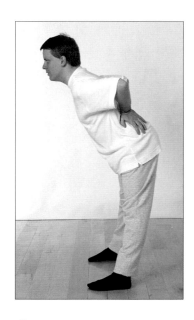 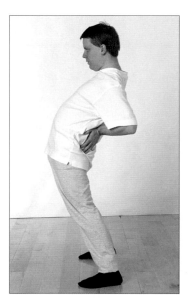

After you have practised for some time near the maximum, come back to the centre in decreasing spirals until you come to a stop. Repeat the exercise in the other direction.

1. Start by standing firmly, with your feet approximately a shoulder-width apart. Lift through the crown of your head, but do not strain. Look forwards.

2. Place the palms of your hands on your kidneys. Start by making small circles with your waist.

3. Gradually increase the size of the circles in an outward spiral. You have reached the maximum when it becomes difficult to keep your head in the same position.

73

Swinging the arms

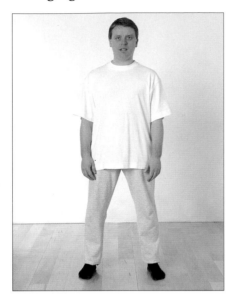

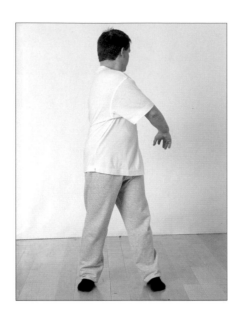

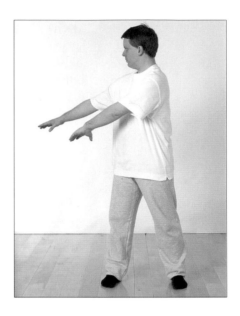

1. Start by standing firmly, with your feet approximately a shoulder-width apart. Lift through the crown of your head, but do not strain. Look forwards.

2. Rotate your body clockwise and anti-clockwise. Allow your arms to hang loosely so that they swing out under their own momentum. Do not simply swing your arms: let your waist become the source of the movement.

3. Gradually increase the amplitude of the movement to increase the benefit of the exercise. Do not overdo the exercise by swinging too hard or stopping suddenly as this can cause injury.

Knee rotation

1. Start by placing your feet next to each other, with no gap between them. Place your hands on your knees to give them a little extra protection. Begin by starting to make small circles that gradually spiral outwards to make bigger circles.

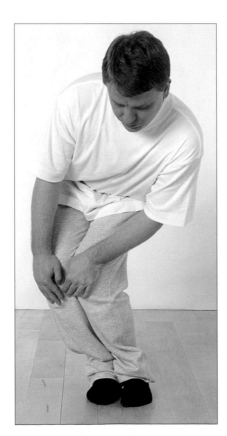

2. When you have done several rotations in one direction, slow down, come back to the centre and repeat in the other direction.

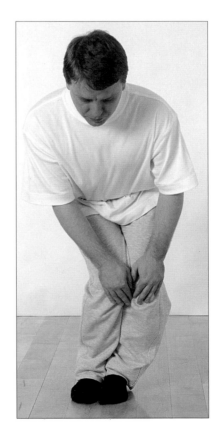

Ankle rotation

Start by touching your big toe on the floor. Make circles with your knee so that your ankle joint is worked in a circular pattern. When you have made several rotations, reverse the direction and then change to the other leg.

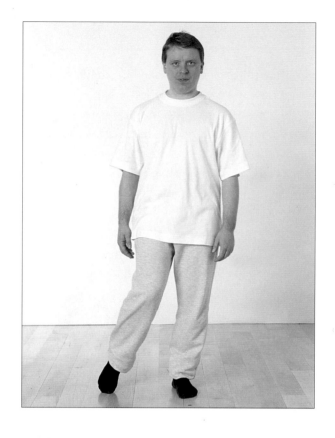

Hamstring stretch

1. Slide your left leg straight backwards and allow your right knee to bend. Rest both hands on your right knee. The intensity of the stretch is determined by how far back you move your left leg. For the best stretch, keep the toes of your left foot pointing as far forward as possible.

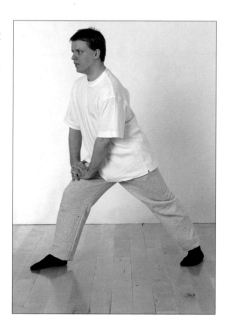

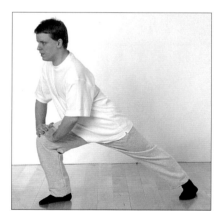

2. Take a deep breath in. On the outward breath, push forwards with your right knee. You will feel the stretches working along the back of your leg if you are performing them correctly. Do not allow your left heel to lift. If you cannot prevent this happening, you are trying to stretch too far. Adjust your position so that you have a shorter stance.

On the inward breath, relax the stance so that the stretch relaxes. Let your knee move back and your body rise. When you have completed ten stretches with your left leg, change stance and do ten stretches with your right leg.

Makkaho stretches

If you want to become supple, you will need to stretch yourself. The rotational exercises are very good for loosening your joints, but you need to stretch your muscles to improve your flexibility. When you stretch your muscles, it would be useful if you could work on specific meridians during the stretch. This would give you a tool both for working on yourself and some 'homework' stretches for your recipients.

Luckily, somebody has already thought of this idea. A common set of stretching exercises taught to Shiatsu students is the Makkaho set. These stretches work all of the classical meridians and the extended meridians that are used in Zen Shiatsu.

The stretches resemble Yoga stretches and the way of using them is similar. You should always stretch on the out breath and relax on the inward breath. Do not bounce as this can cause injury. Do not attempt a deep stretch unless you are warmed up, and

know your own limits. The most important rule for stretching is: **if it hurts, stop!** Pain tells you that you are going too far. Over-zealous stretching can do more harm than good.

When you are coming out of a stretch, always come out the same way that you went into it. A good example is the stomach/spleen stretch. If you get your back all of the way down to the floor for the stretch, do not injure yourself by trying to sit up again in one go. Use the same steps that you used to go into the stretch and you will avoid injury.

There is also a visualisation aspect to the exercises. On the outward breath, imagine that you are breathing out a negative aspect of the element that you are stretching and, on the inward breath, breathe in the positive aspect of the energy. The aspects are shown below and will help you to involve your mind with the stretch, rather than just your body.

Element	Negative (out breath)	Positive (in breath)
Metal	Grief	Courage
Earth	Worry	Serenity
Water	Fear	Gentleness
Fire	Arrogance	Love
Wood	Anger	Kindness

The metal stretch

This metal-stretch exercise stretches the lung and large-intestine meridians. Viewed from the front, it resembles the letter 'A'.

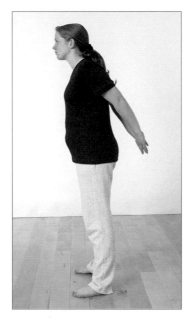 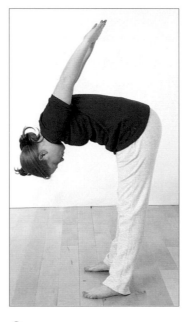 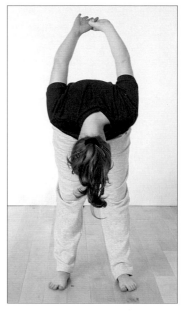

$1.$ Stand with your feet a shoulder-width apart and link your thumbs behind your back.

$2.$ On an outward breath, bend your body forwards. Work with the stretch for a few breaths before coming out of it.

$3.$ Come out of the stretch on an outward breath. Do this by pushing your hands forwards and letting your body follow them.

The earth stretch

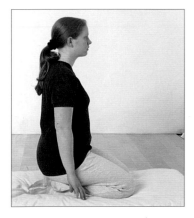 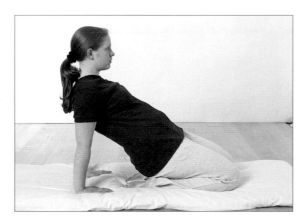 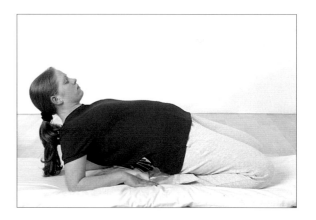

This stretches the stomach and spleen meridians. Viewed from the side, it resembles the letter 'B'.

$1.$ Kneel on the floor.

$2.$ Breath out and lean back onto your hands. (This may be as far as your body will stretch for now; if it feels like a big enough stretch, hold it for two or three breaths and come out of it.)

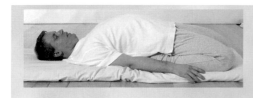

If you still have plenty of room left to stretch, breathe out and lower your back to the floor.

When coming out of the stretch, be sure to go through the stage where you put your elbows on the floor. Otherwise you will strain your back.

The fire stretch

This stretch works with the heart and small-intestine meridians. It resembles the letter 'C' when viewed from the side.

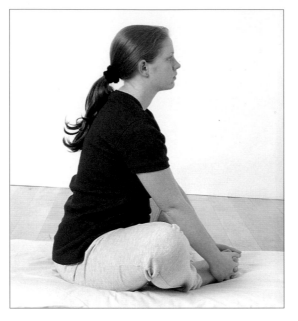

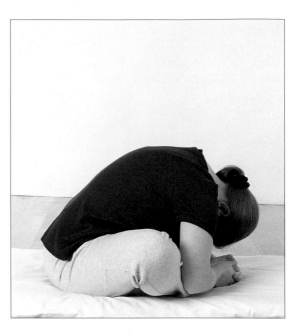

1. Sit with the soles of your feet together and draw them as close to your groin as you can. Grab your feet with your hands and keep your elbows outside your shins.

2. On an outward breath, bend your body forwards and release your neck.

The water stretch

This stretch will work the bladder and kidney meridians. From the side, it resembles the letter 'D'.

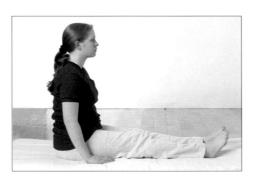

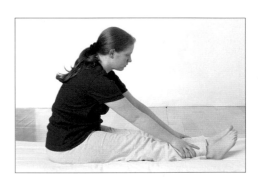

1. Sit with your legs out and your back straight.

2. On an exhalation, bend forwards and grab your ankles.

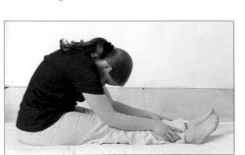

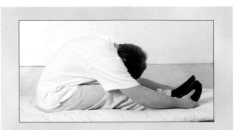

3. Increase the stretch by dropping your elbows and releasing your neck.

If you are able, repeat the stretch, this time bending forwards and grabbing kidney point 1, on the middle of the foot.

The secondary fire stretch

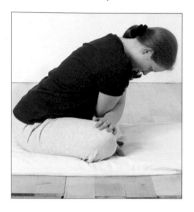

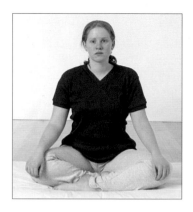

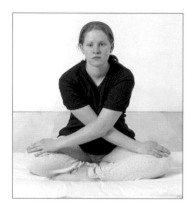

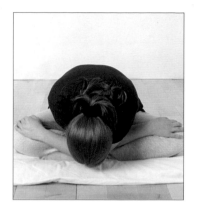

This stretch works the heart-protector and triple-heater meridians. From the side, it resembles the letter 'E'.

1. Sit with your legs crossed in front of you.

2. Cross your arms and touch your knees. If your left shin is at the front, your left forearm should be in front of the right.

3. Exhale and lean forwards. Press on your knees to open your groin.

Repeat, crossing your legs the other way.

The wood stretch

This stretch will work the gall-bladder and liver meridians. When viewed from the front, it resembles the letter 'F'.

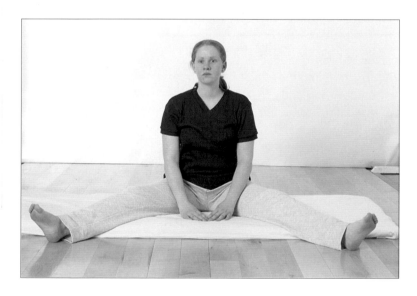

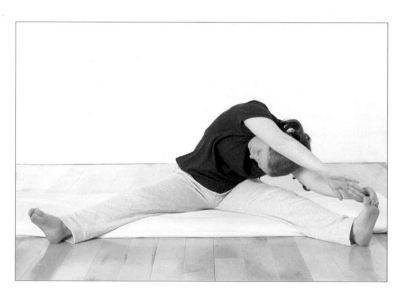

1. Sit with your legs fairly far apart. (Do not stretch your legs so widely that you cannot execute the stretch for your upper body.) Keep your back straight.

2. Exhale and lean to one side. If you can reach, grab liver point 1 on your big toe with the hand that reaches over your head. With your other hand, grab gall-bladder point 44. If this is not yet a possibility, just grab your ankle. Do not collapse your Hara.

Grounding exercise

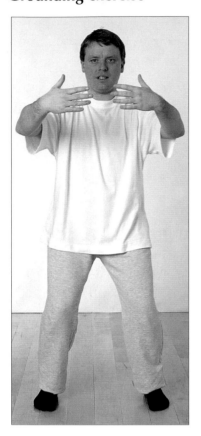

We have already spoken of the fact that effective Shiatsu needs to be grounded. The following exercise is very helpful for improving your sense of grounding. It is called 'standing like a tree' because you need to imagine that a root extends into the earth from your feet and that you are growing upwards like a tree.

Try practising it for a small amount of time each day and gradually build up the time to fifteen or twenty minutes. You will soon feel the difference.

Start with your feet a shoulder-width apart and parallel. Keep your back straight, your head upright, your eyes alert, but not fixed, and relax your breathing.

Bend your knees slightly as though you were resting your buttocks on the edge of a table. Keep your head up and your back straight.

Bring up your arms in front of your chest as shown. Do not raise your shoulders, and try to stay relaxed.

Hold the position for as long as is comfortable. Keep your breathing gentle and relaxed.

Hara meditation

The following routine is not a complicated one. It is intended to be something that you can practise at virtually any time and in any place whenever your have a few spare minutes. Start with learning how to breathe into your Hara until it becomes natural. When you can do this easily, try the meditation and feel the energy moving.

Hara breathing
When learning how to breathe into the Hara, try to pick places that have a natural vibrancy, or energy, of their own. This will mean that the energy is flowing around the area and that the Ki is not stagnant. You will naturally relax your body and mind, so make sure that you will not be discomforted by cold.

Sit in the Seiza position. Close your eyes and relax your mind. Breathe into the Hara by expanding it on an inhalation and contracting it on an exhalation. Keep the movement gentle and do not force it. Observe the rhythm of the Hara. Let your body and mind relax.

Place your hands on your Tan Tien point, just below the navel. Feel your hands moving on the Hara as you breathe in and out.

When you have finished, rub your hands over your Hara in a circular fashion.

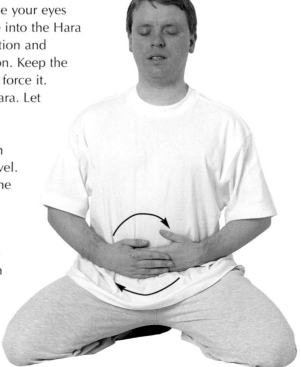

Feeling energy

Many people believe that there must be something beneficial in Shiatsu, but cannot accept the idea that energy is involved, simply because they cannot see it. Apart from some highly developed individuals who can actually see auras and Kirlian photographs, our energy is invisible. Just because you cannot see energy does not mean that you cannot feel it, however. To deny the existence of energy after you have felt it would be like denying the existence of electricity after you have had an electric shock!

The following exercise is simple and teaches you what energy feels like. Do not be fooled by its simplicity. When you are trying to feel a meridian, and to move the energy within it, this is the type of feeling that you are aiming for.

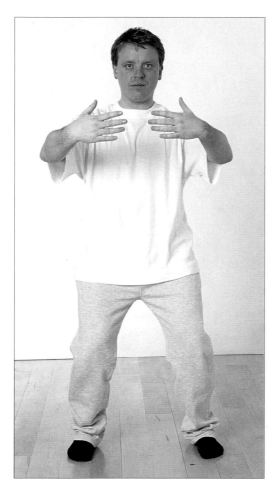

1. Start with the 'standing like a tree' exercise or Hara breathing. This is simply to get you tuned into the energy. If you are already quite sensitive, you may not need to do this.

2. Turn the palms of your hands inwards, facing towards each other. Keep your shoulders down and your arms relaxed. Gradually move your hands towards each other. At a certain point, you should pick up a sensation that feels like an invisible force, or heat, in the gap between your hands. Play with this feeling and see if you can make the 'energy ball' between your hands bigger.

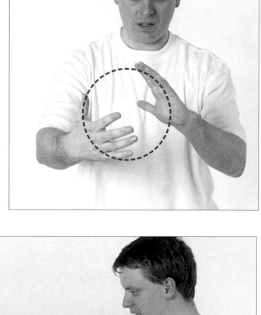

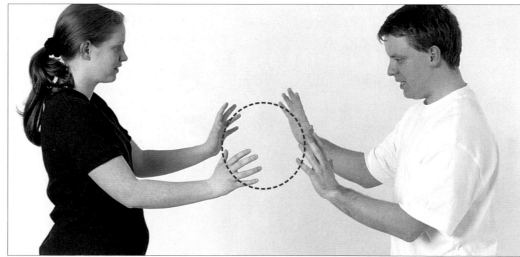

3. If you have a friend nearby who has been doing the same, face each other and make an energy ball between you. Try to feel its shape. Notice how the feeling changes if your friend walks away.

Basic Shiatsu techniques

Before considering what you are actually going to do with your Shiatsu, it is worth thinking about where you are going to practise it. You will ideally need a room that is fairly warm and airy. It needs to be warm because relaxation may make your recipient feel cold. It is also a good idea to have a few blankets handy to wrap the recipient in if they feel cold.

Fresh air is always good: it creates a pleasant atmosphere and helps to disperse stagnant Ki. For this reason, it is a good idea never to allow smoking in the area that you use for Shiatsu. Try to arrange your space so that when you work around the recipient you are not constantly banging into furniture.

The best work surface is a futon mattress. This will make the recipient feel more comfortable when lying on the floor. Try to find the biggest one you can. This is because you will be kneeling on it for some time and it will protect your knees. You will also need some cushions or pillows. These will support different parts of the recipient's body, such as the head when they are in the side position.

It is also a good idea to have some easily washable, cotton cloths for the recipient to lay their head on. This is hygienic practice and may

save the recipient from potential embarrassment: when you are lying face down, having your bladder meridian worked on, it is easy to become so relaxed that you dribble from your mouth.

The recipient should be wearing loose, easy-fitting clothes and no shoes. As the therapist, you will need the same basic outfit. White is commonly worn because this is the colour that reflects all of the other energies, in the same way that it reflects light.

We will now consider some of the basic techniques used in Shiatsu. There are many techniques used by Shiatsu professionals, but these three provide the basic skills that you will require to give a treatment.

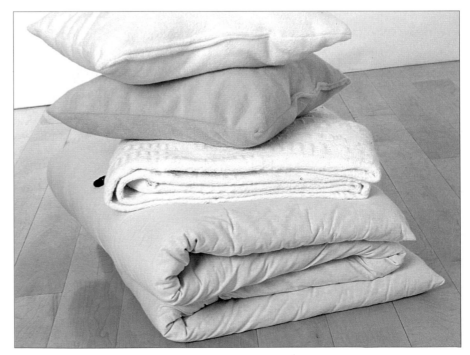

Always think of your own comfort, as well as your client's.

82

Stretching

Stretching is a useful technique in Shiatsu that has many benefits, such as improving the circulation of the blood and lymphatic fluid, improving mobility and bringing the meridian channels to the surface. To avoid injuring your recipient, you must be sensitive to their needs. It is a good idea to watch their face if you can: you will soon see if you are hurting them (remember that they will not always tell you).

It also helps to understand some of the science behind stretching. The first thing to remember is that a muscle fibre cannot actually change its length. Because a muscle is naturally in a state of contraction, the way to increase its mobility is to reduce the amount of contracting tension on the muscle. Ligaments do not stretch at all under normal conditions. If you stretch a ligament, you will cause a serious injury.

When you stretch a muscle, it should be done slowly. This allows you to overcome the stretch reflex and be sensitive. Make sure that the recipient is breathing in a relaxed way. Some people tend to hold their breath when they stretch, which is detrimental.

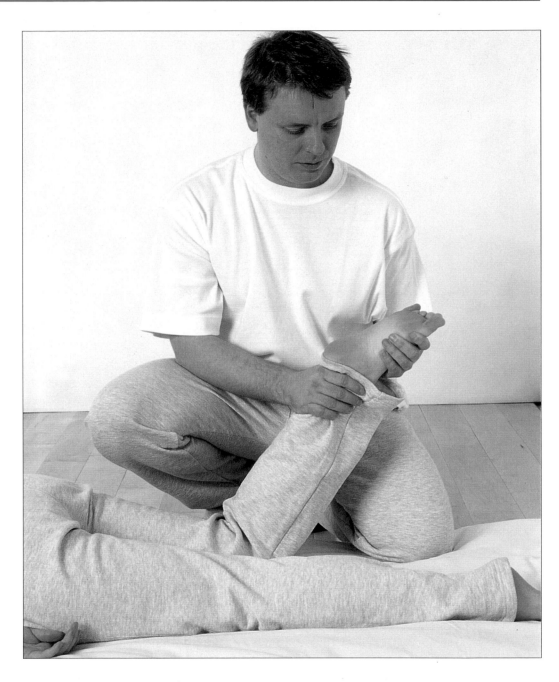

1. The recipient should be lying face down on the mat. Take hold of their foot and ankle.

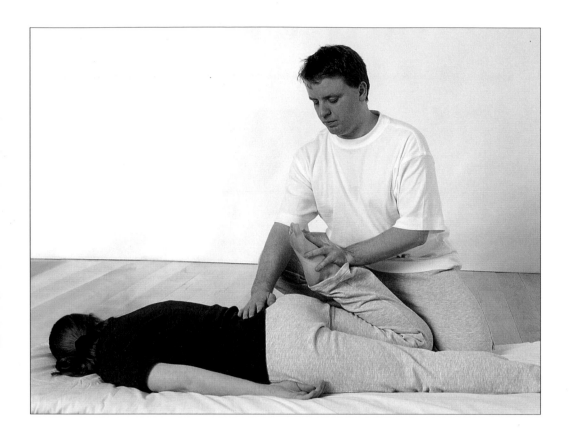

2. Listen to the recipient's breathing. On their exhalation, push their foot towards their buttock to stretch their leg.

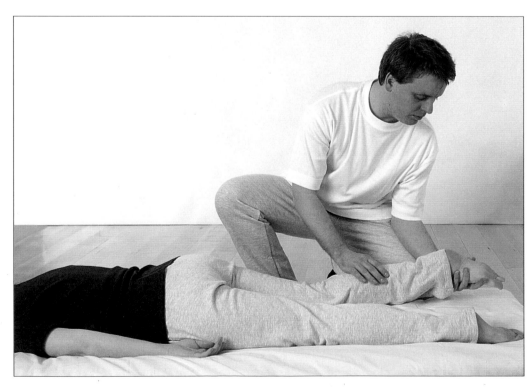

3. When you have finished the stretch, be sure to replace their leg on the mat – do not simply drop it.

A holding technique

Another simple and effective technique is holding. One of the basic ideas of Shiatsu is that of support, and holding is a way of giving support.

The recipient needs to be lying on their back. Make sure that there is not a light above their eyes or they will never relax.

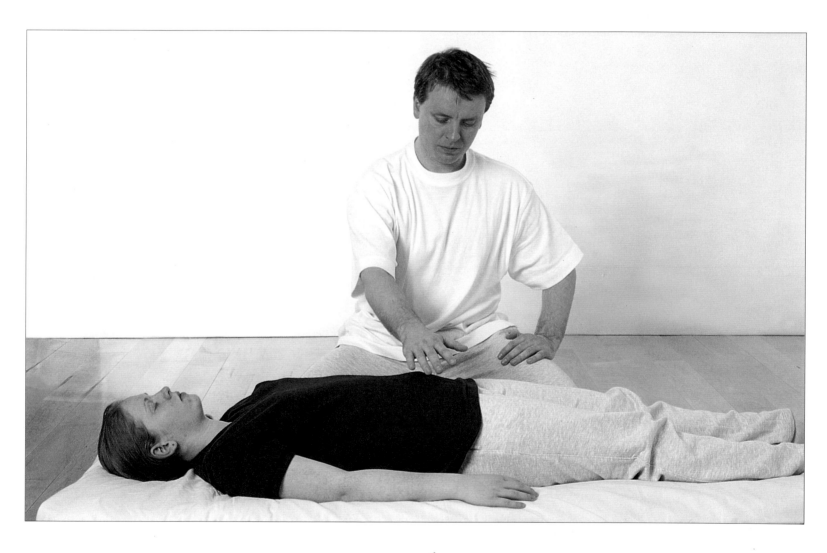

1. Remember the exercise that we did for feeling energy. Using the same sensitivity, hold your hand above the recipient's Hara and feel the energy.

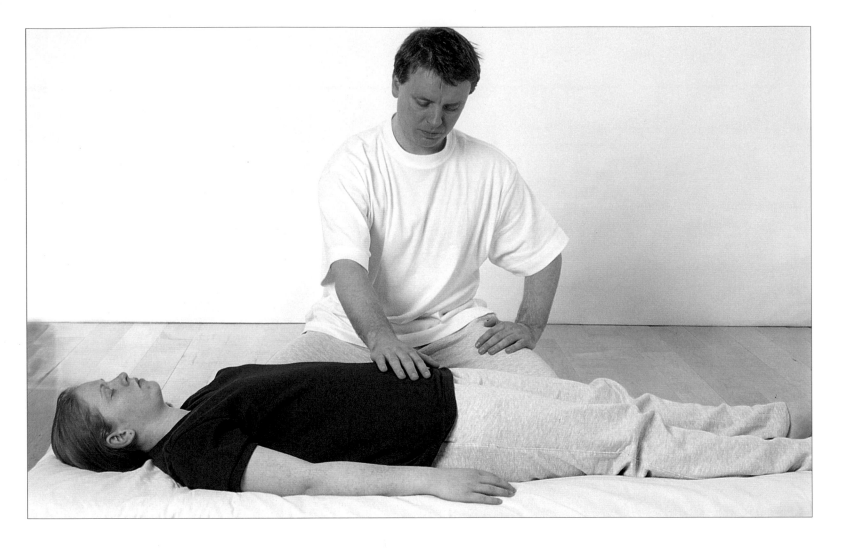

2. Let your hand slowly and gently float downwards. Be sensitive to the movements of the energy and follow them. When your hand has found its path to the place where you can touch the physical Hara, gently place it on their abdomen. The pressure should be light so that you can maintain sensitivity.

As the recipient breathes in and out, your hand should float up and down on the Hara like a cork on the sea. Tune into the recipient's breathing and go with the movements of their Hara – do not try to control it for this technique.

When you think that you have done all that you can (usually after five minutes or more), remove your hand. Do this by waiting for the Hara to rise, but then do not move your hand down with it. If you are gentle, the recipient normally thinks that your hand is still on them for a few minutes after you remove it.

Thumb pressure

Shiatsu uses thumbs, hands, elbows, knees and feet to apply pressure. The most commonly used of these is the thumb, which we shall discuss here.

Generally, the following things need to be understood.

- Stay connected with the energy; do not just dig your thumbs into the recipient.
- When working with a Tsubo, you need to be at a right angle to it to achieve the best results.
- If you work in a gentle way, it is easier for you to be sensitive to the energy.
- Remember to look after your own thumbs! I have seen therapists who have suffered from joint problems in their thumbs as a result of applying too much pressure.

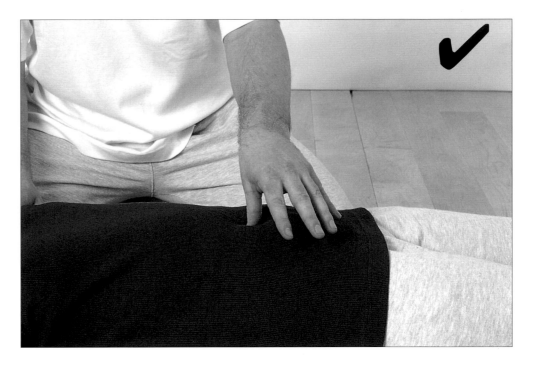

Correct: the thumb should always be held at a right angle.

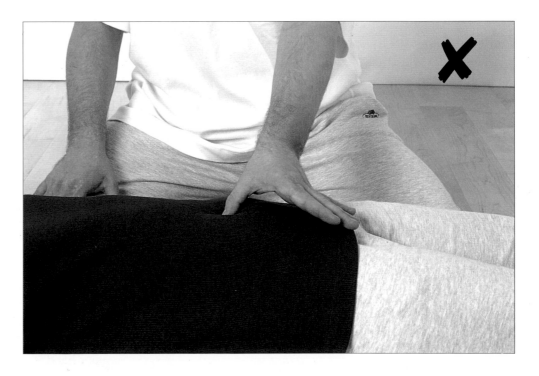

Incorrect: the thumb should not be bent.

Learn one good technique

In some traditional styles of Karate, you will start by learning one technique – perhaps a punch. Before you are allowed to learn other techniques, you must master that punch. By the time that your master teaches you other techniques, such as blocking, you will have perfected one technique and will have learned much about how the body works.

For example, what originally seemed a simple hand movement will now involve the whole of your body and paying attention to your Hara. This will mean that you will learn the other techniques very quickly and that the training will have paid off.

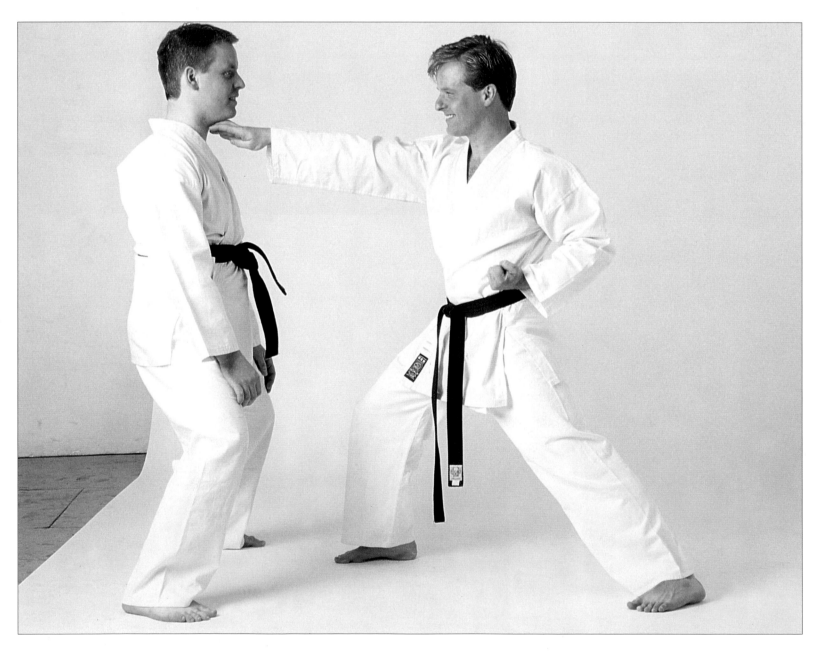

One good technique is more valuable than several bad ones.

Shiatsu technique is the same. There is great value in learning how to perform one technique well rather than a variety of poor ones. An example here is the stretch. If you learn all about muscle dynamics, meridian locations and how to move with your client to perform the stretch and do it well, you will have learned much.

If you then want to extend your knowledge into knowledge of Tsubos and their effects, you will already have a good base knowledge to work from.

This approach involves investing time and effort at the beginning and reaping the benefits later on. Always remember that we are all constantly learning, so it is good to use this idea to give you a focus.

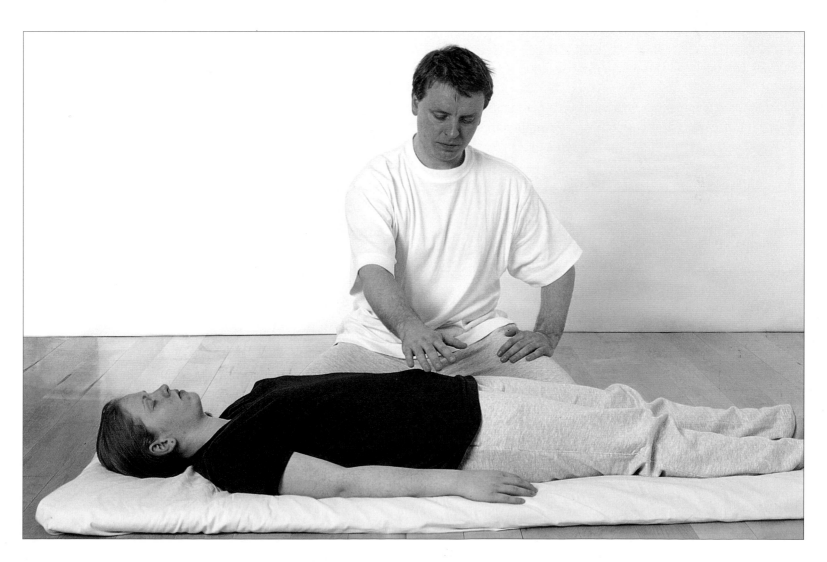

Shiatsu procedures

Learning Shiatsu is analogous to learning how to play jazz. The aim of a jazz musician is to be able to play free-form music. This means that the musician will not need a specific tune to play: he will respond to the rest of the band and the audience and will try to play his best tune. The jazz musician will not try to analyse his music, but will go with the flow.

Good Shiatsu is similar. In the case of Shiatsu, the flow that we follow is sometimes called the Tao. Like the musician, the healer does not instantly know how to improvise. The healer has to learn some set routines, just as the musician learns set tunes. When you have the tune inside you, you can play with it, but first you need to learn the tune.

The following routines are only four out of many that you could learn. They use the basic positions of lying in the prone, supine and side positions, finishing with the sitting position. When you have practised the routines, feel free to add or subtract anything that you like. If you can work in the four positions, you will be able to give a treatment.

Finally, do not be too concerned about getting things wrong. If you make a mistake, just carry on as if you had not made it. As long as you remain sensitive and gentle, you will not harm anyone. If you stop and begin again, it will break the flow. As the rock guitarist Jeff Beck once said, 'Things turn out better by accident sometimes'. But you can't arrange accidents.

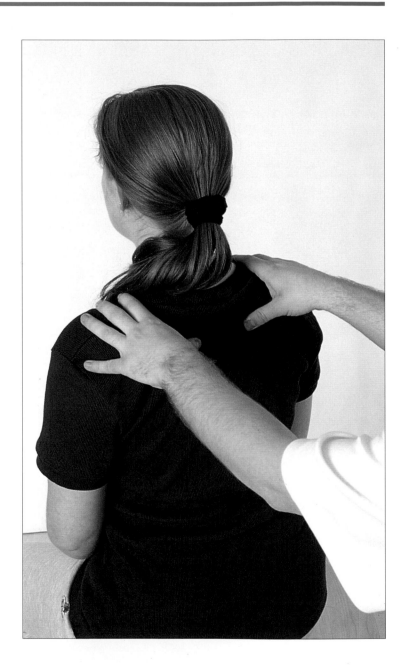

Working in the prone, or face-down, position

This routine should take about twenty to thirty minutes to perform

Cat-walking

When a cat walks, it stays relaxed and natural. In this warming-up technique for the recipient, you will walk your hands over the recipient's back, buttocks, arms and legs. There is no particular sequence, just keep your palm relaxed and use them to massage the whole of your recipient's body, as shown in the illustrations. It will relax the client and help you to establish contact with them.

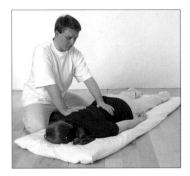
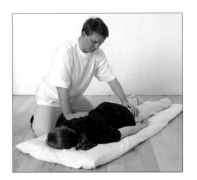
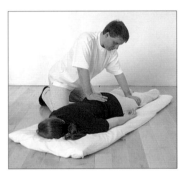
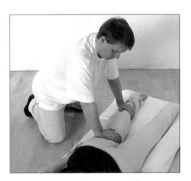

Cross stretches

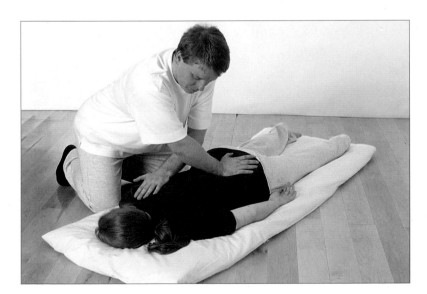
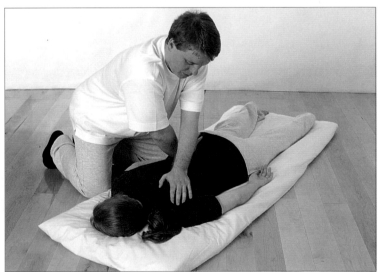

1. Cross your forearms to form an 'X' shape. Place one hand low on the back, near to the buttocks, and the other near to the shoulder blade. Gently lower your weight so that your hands are forced apart to perform a cross stretch.

2. Repeat on the other diagonal.

Lateral stretches

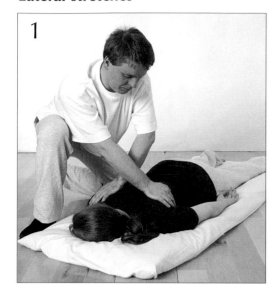

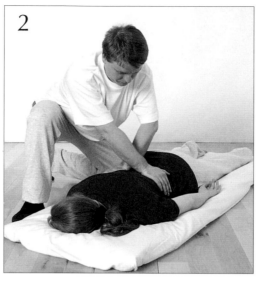

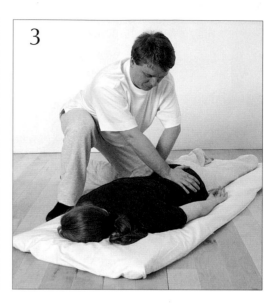

Form an 'X' shape with your arms. Place your hands on either side of the spine and stretch the back laterally, beginning at the shoulders (1), working through the waist (2) and then down to the base of the spine (3).

Wave-rocking

When you work on someone's back, you will be working with the bladder channel, which is ruled by the water element. Keep this idea in your mind when rocking.

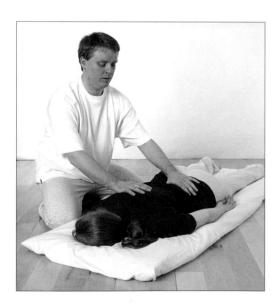

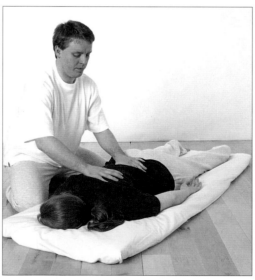

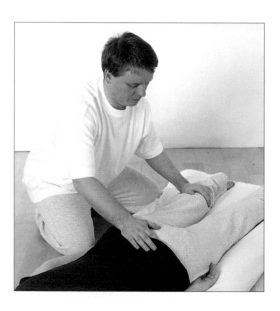

1. Use one hand to start the mid-part of the back moving.

2. When the mid-section is moving freely, use the other hand to rock other parts of the body. If done gently, it will relax the recipient.

3. You can also use this technique to rock the legs.

Sacral rub

Finish this part of the sequence by giving the recipient's sacrum a massage to try to mobilise it. Remember to keep your pace gentle and steady.

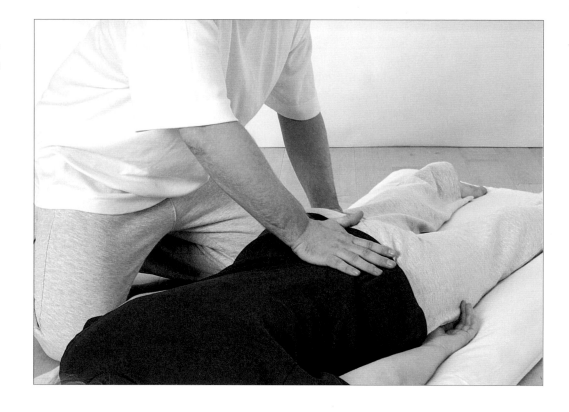

Back rub

$1.$ Keep one hand on the recipient and move around to their head. Try not to lose contact.

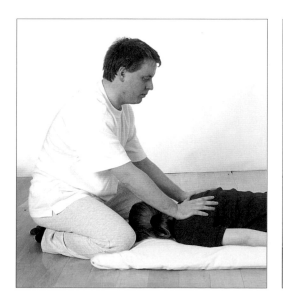

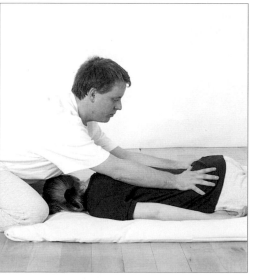

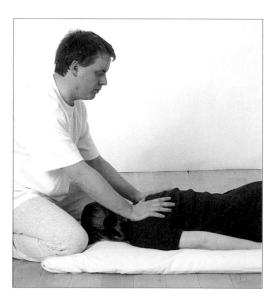

$2.$ Now rub down the length of their back with the heels of your hands.

$3.$ When you reach the sacrum, stop and rock it a little to loosen the back.

$4.$ Walk your hands back up their body and repeat two to three times.

Thumb the bladder meridian

We are now going to work both sides of the bladder meridian. If you are unsure about the location, just remember that it is either side of the spine and the width of two fingers away from it. The Tsubos are in the gaps between the ribs.

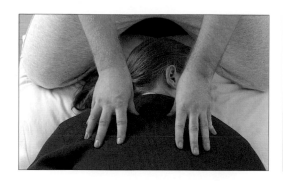

1. Start by gently pressing your thumbs into the points at the top of the spine. This is point number 11 on the bladder meridian. Gradually work through the points.

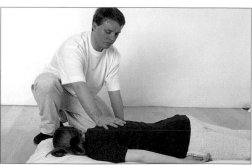

2. When you reach somewhere around points 16 or 17, you will have just about come to the end of your reach. Remember to keep your thumbs perpendicular to recipient's back.

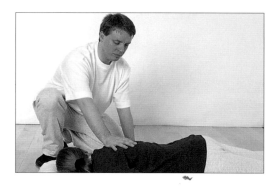

3. You will now need to move to continue working. Keep contact with the recipient's body as you move.

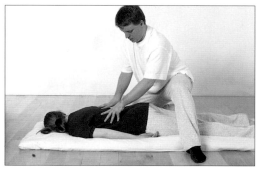

4. Move around to the side of the recipient to work the rest of the back until you have worked the sacrum.

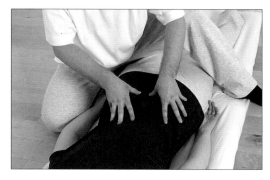

5. It is important to hold your hands correctly when working the points.

Palm down the leg

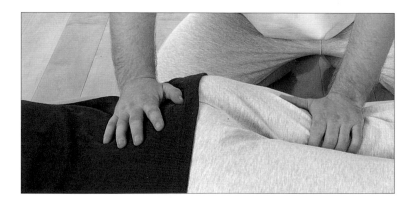

1. Keep one hand on the sacrum and use the other hand to palm down your client's leg.

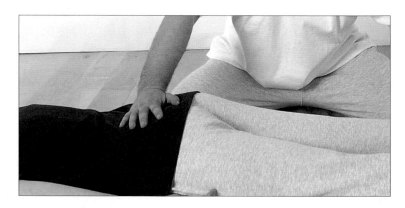

2. Continue until you have worked all the way from the top of the leg to the bottom.

Leg stretches

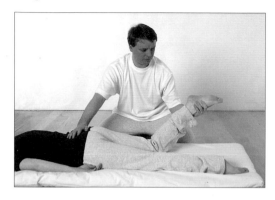

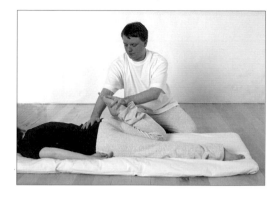

$1.$ Leave your passive hand on the sacrum and grab the ankle with the other.

$2.$ Carefully pull the foot towards the buttock to stretch the leg.

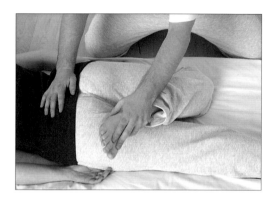

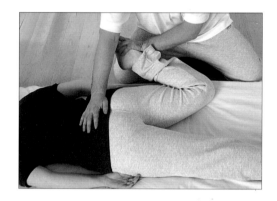

$3.$ You can also pull the foot to the left of the recipient's body.

$4.$ To balance this move, you should also stretch the leg to the right.

When you have finished, put the leg down very carefully – do not drop it.

Thumb down the bladder meridian in the leg

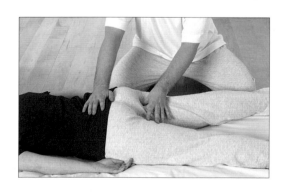

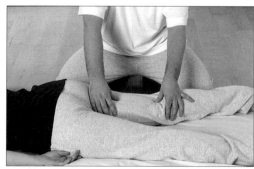

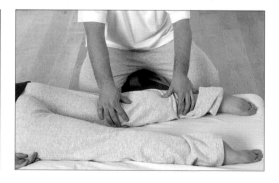

$1.$ Still with your passive hand on the sacrum, work your thumb down the bladder meridian in the centre of the leg. Imagine that an energetic circuit is being made between your active and passive hands.

$2.$ When your active hand has moved too far away from the passive hand for your comfort, move the passive hand further down the bladder meridian. Try to place it over one of the Tsubos, such as bladder point 37.

$3.$ Continue in this way until you reach the ankle.

Ankle rotation

Hold the lower leg with one hand and rotate the foot with the other to loosen the ankle.

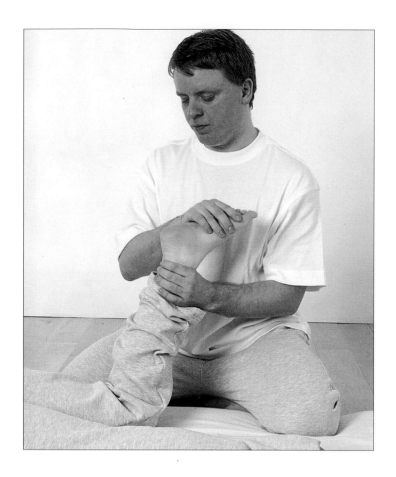

Work the bladder meridian in the foot

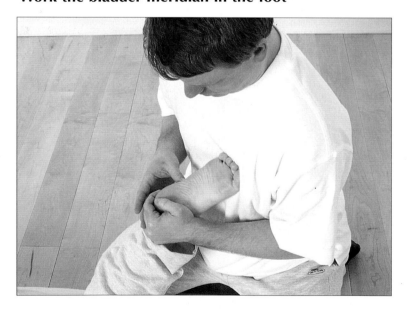

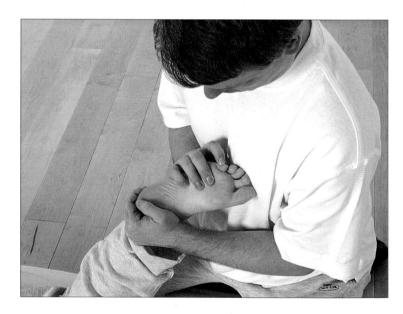

1. Hold bladder point 60 with one hand and then work through the foot.

2. Continue working down the foot until you reach point 67 on the little toe.

When you have finished, put the foot down gently.

Work the other leg

Move to the other side of the person to that which you have been working on and repeat the procedure on the other leg.

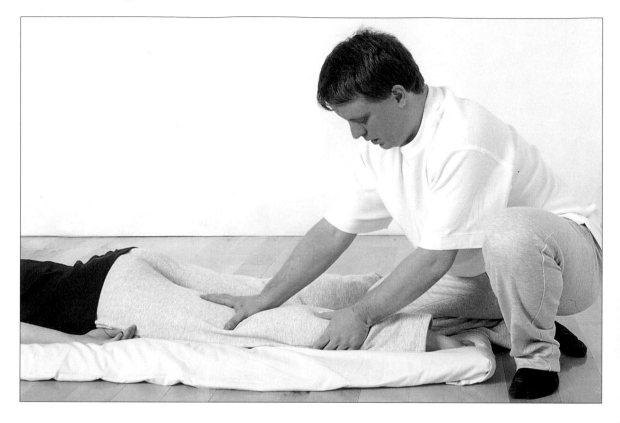

Hold kidney point 1

Finish the treatment by holding kidney point 1, in the middle of the feet, for a minute or so.

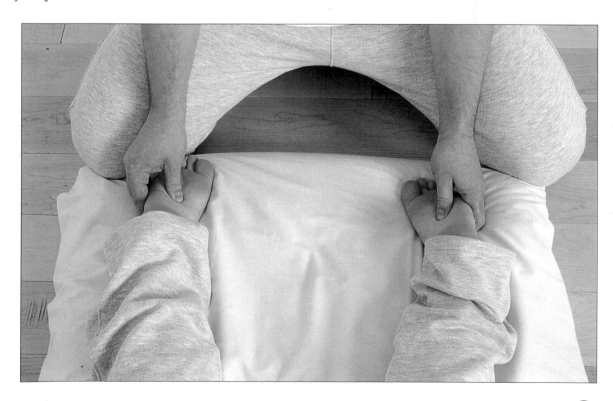

Working in the supine, or face-up, position

Your client may be more comfortable if you give them a small pillow for
their head. The supine position is ideal for working with earth energy in
the stomach and spleen meridians, so these will be described. Hara work
is briefly described, as this is very centring, which is another feature of
earth energy. This should take twenty to twenty-five minutes.

Pull the heels to stretch the legs

Hold the heels and sink
back into a squatting
position to give a gentle pull
on the legs. Do not pull so
hard that your client thinks
that they are being dragged
across the floor.

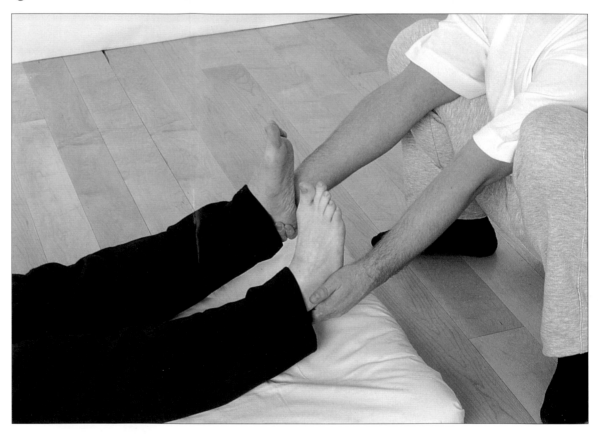

Shake the legs

Produce a gentle shaking movement from your Hara and use it to shake
the legs. Place the feet down gently afterwards.

Knee to chest

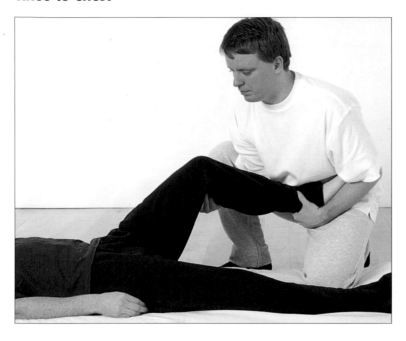

1. Pick up one leg gently and begin to push the knee towards the chest.

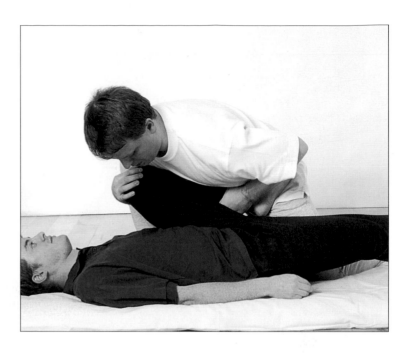

2. This will stretch the gluteal muscles and the lower back. Use your body weight to power the stretch.

Hip rotations

Keep the knee bent and hold it close to your body. Rotate from your Hara to open and rotate the hip joint.

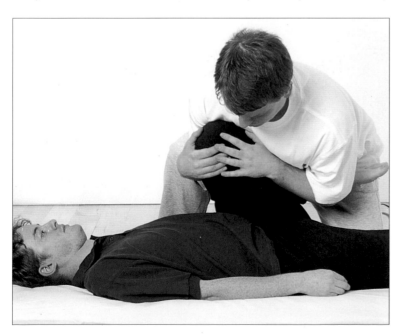

1. First rotate the knee to the right of the recipient's body.

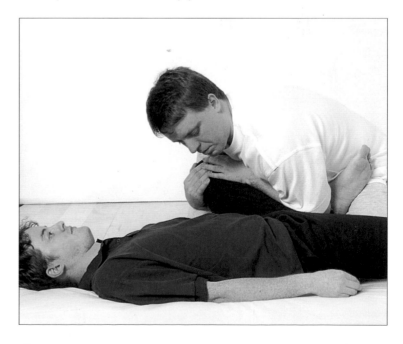

2. Then rotate the knee to the left of the body.

Ankle rotations

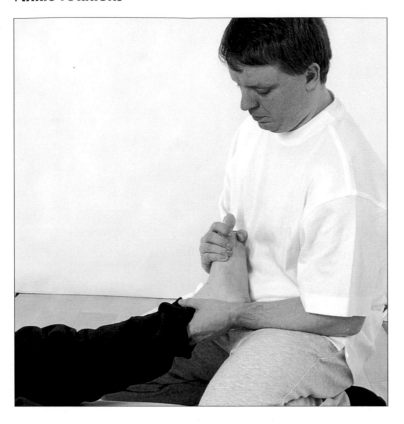

Bring the foot back to the outstretched position and then rotate the ankle.

Work the other leg

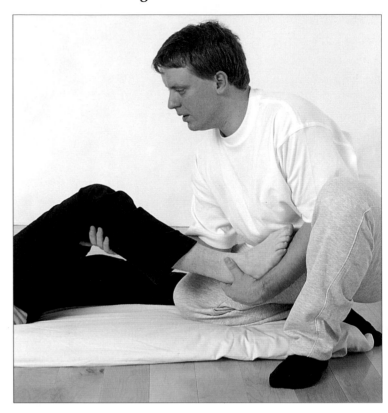

Repeat the procedure for the other leg.

Massage the hand

Move around to a position in which you can pick up the recipient's hand comfortably.

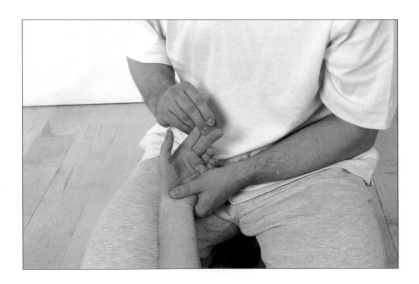

1. First massage the fingers gently.

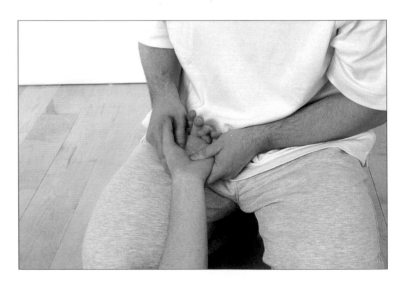

2. Then move on to massage the whole hand.

Palm down the arm

Gently use your body weight to palm down your client's arm, as in the cat-walking-for-the-back treatment

Repeat the procedure for the other arm.

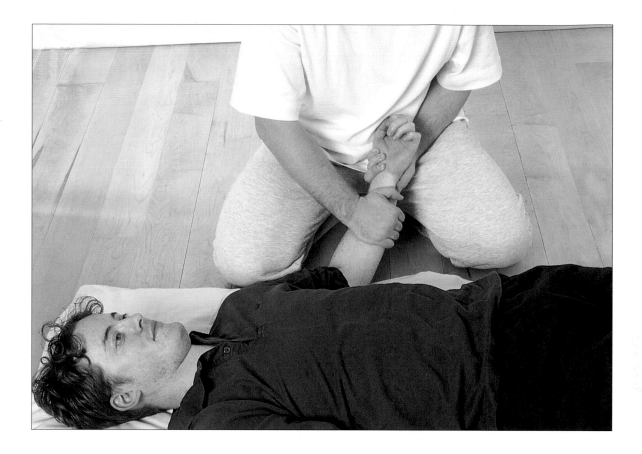

Work the Hara

A simple and effective way of working with the Hara is to use both hands to spiral on the Hara in a clockwise direction. When you have completed several spirals, use your hands to smooth across the Hara as if you were smoothing down the icing on a cake.

This would be a reasonable point at which to stop the treatment if you so desired. It would also be a good point at which to work the stomach and spleen meridians.

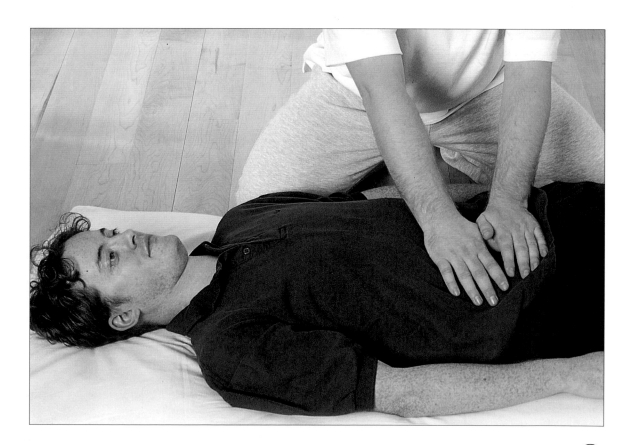

Work the spleen meridian in the foot, shin and knee

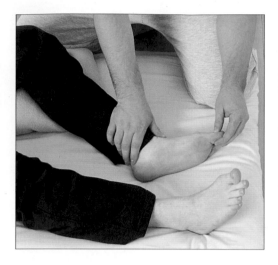 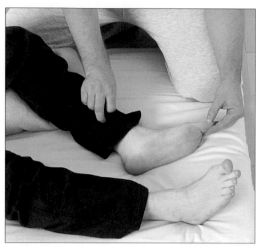 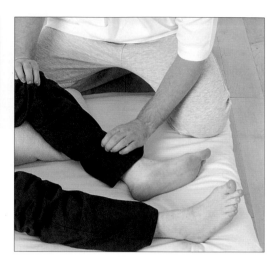

1. Hold the spleen point 1 at the end of the big toe with one hand and work down to spleen point 6 with the other. Place a cushion under the knee for extra comfort.

2. When you reach spleen point 6 with your active hand, move the passive hand down to take its place.

3. This will make it easier to work up to the knee.

Work the spleen meridian on the inner thigh

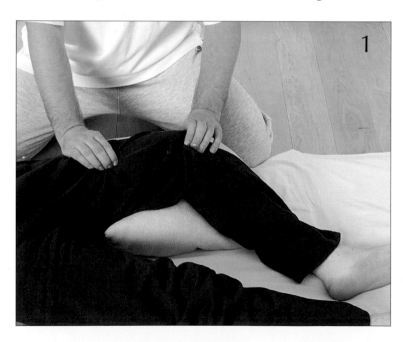 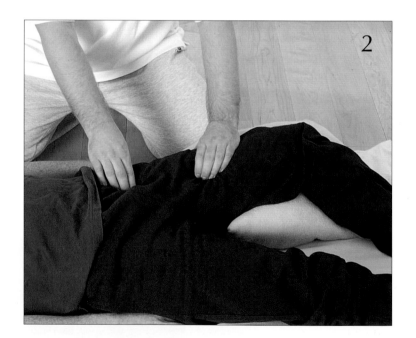

Keep hold of spleen point 10 and work up to the Hara, as shown in illustrations 1 and 2.

Work the spleen meridian through the Hara

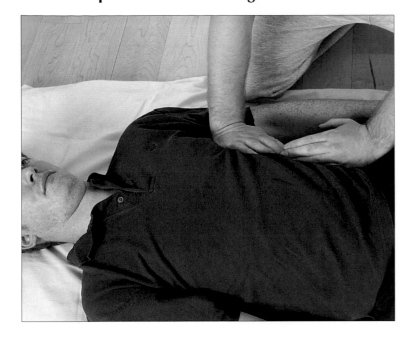

Gently work the spleen meridian through the Hara. It is approximately one hand's-width away from the centre line. Go as far as the bottom of the ribcage. This is a reasonable place to stop working the meridian.

Work the stomach meridian through the Hara

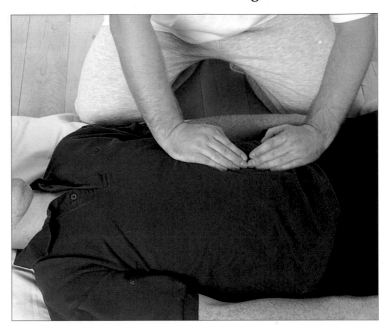

The stomach meridian lies on a line that is 2 cun (just over 2 finger-widths) away from the centre line. Work along this line until you are approximately level with the trouser line.

Work the spleen meridian in the foot, shin and knee

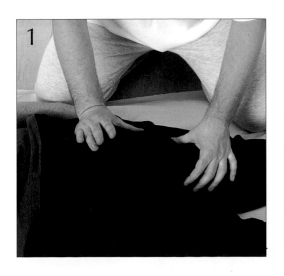

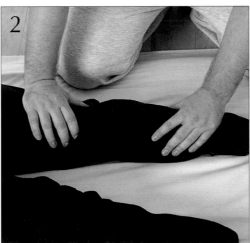

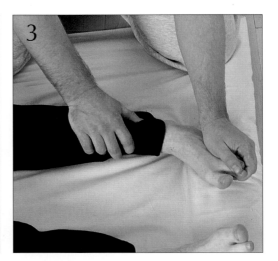

The stomach meridian is on the outer side of the leg. Work through the meridian in the same way that you did for the spleen meridian. Pay special attention to points 34 (1), 36 (2) and 40 (3), if you can remember where they are.

Finish this part of the treatment by holding stomach point 45, on the end of the second toe, for a few minutes.

Finish the treatment by working the stomach and spleen meridians on the other side of the body.

Working in the side position

The side position is ideal for working with wood energy in the gall-bladder and liver meridians. The recipient should be in the recovery position of basic first-aid practice. This makes them more stable for you to work on and therefore also more comfortable.

Make sure that you have enough cushions or pillows to support the neck. The treatment normally takes about fifteen minutes for each side of the body.

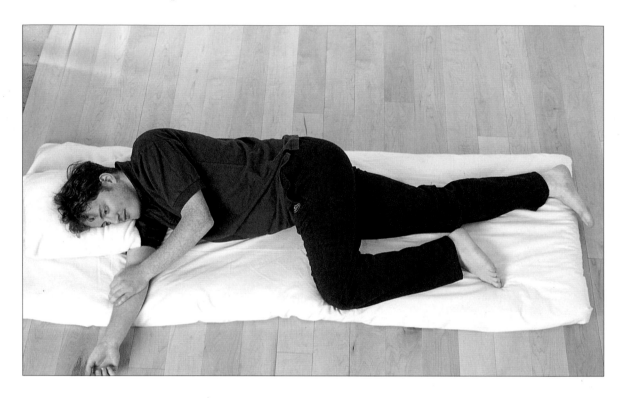

Shoulder rotations

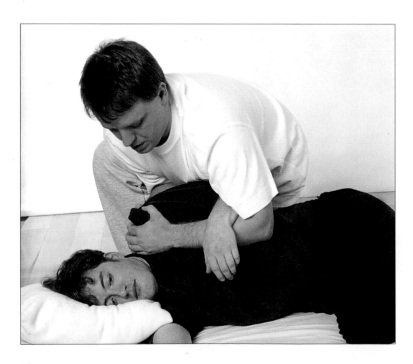

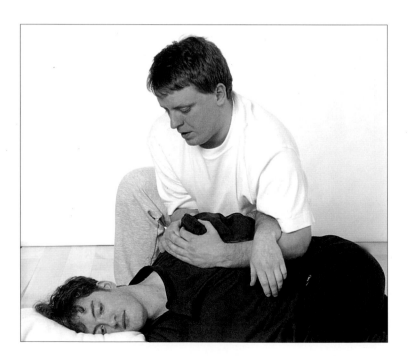

1. Put both of your hands over the shoulder and rotate the shoulder. Keep close to your client for maximum body contact and work from your Hara.

2. Start with small rotations and gradually enlarge them.

Shoulder pull

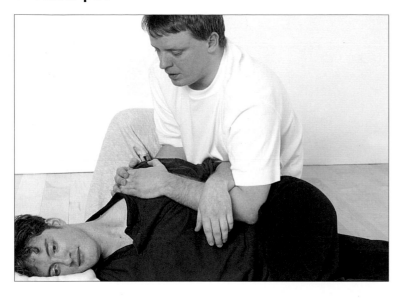

1. Keep both hands in contact with the shoulder and lean back to stretch the shoulder and neck.

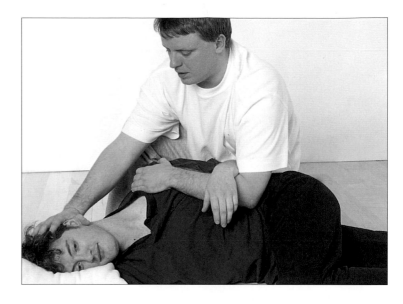

2. Let go with one hand and place the thumb on gall-bladder point 12, below the ear. Move the hand that is on the shoulder up slightly so that you can place a finger on gall-bladder point 21. Stretch the side of the neck by pulling on these points.

Arm stretch (vertical)

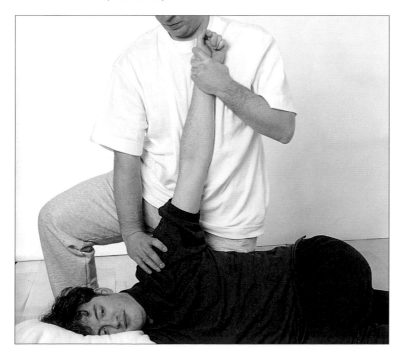

Grab the wrist and pull the arm vertically upwards for a stretch. This is a good opportunity quickly to work the heart-protector channel in the middle of the arm.

Arm stretch (horizontal)

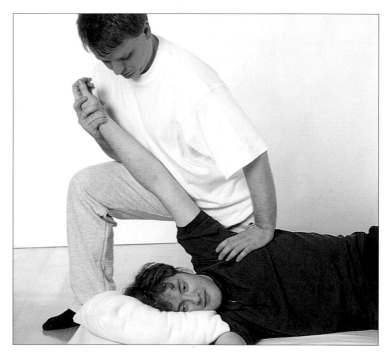

Keep hold of the arm and lift it past the ear for another stretch. Use your body to lunge forwards when you do this.

Palm the lung meridian

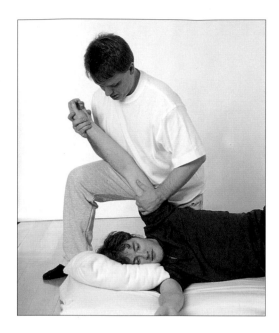

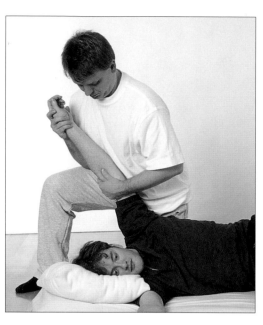

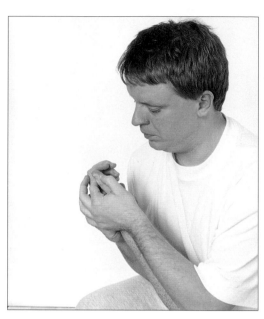

1. The lung meridian is now exposed, so start at lung point 1 on the chest.

2. Work down the arm, along the meridian.

3. Finish at the end point on the thumb.

'Chicken-wing' stretch

The reason for the name of this stretch is obvious when you see it being done.

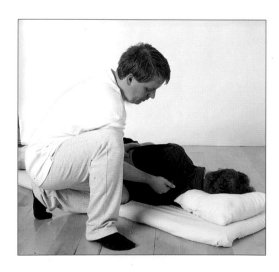

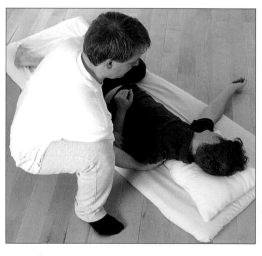

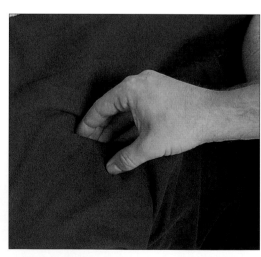

1. Bring the elbow back so that the scapula protrudes.

2. Place your fingers under the scapula and pull the arm back to help to mobilise the scapula.

3. This photograph shows the hand movement clearly.

General meridian work

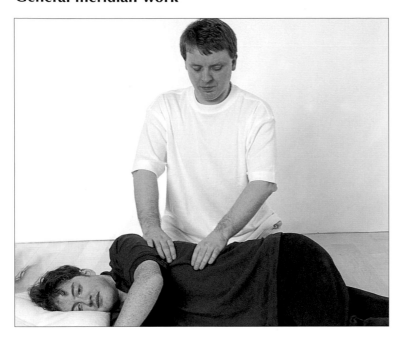

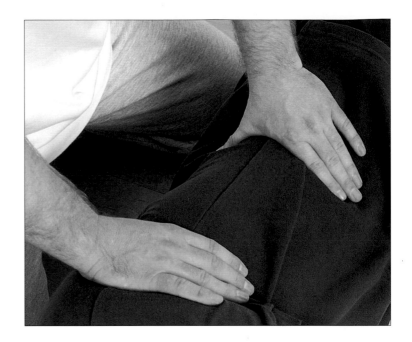

1. This technique uses the webbing between your finger and your thumb.

2. Work down the gall-bladder meridian in the side of the recipient's body. Keep the idea of wood energy in your head because you are using intent rather than aiming for specific points.

Side stretch

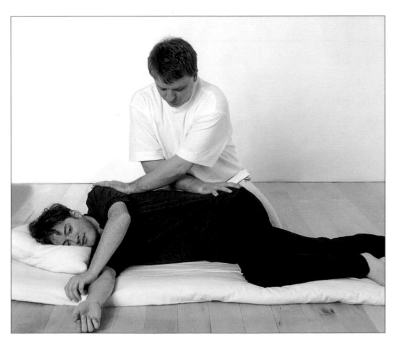

Use both hands to stretch along the side of the recipient's body.

Work gall-bladder point 30

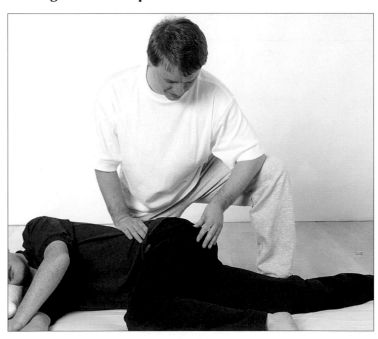

Lift the recipient's knee to a high position to expose gall-bladder point 30, which you can work with your thumb. Supporting your elbow with your knee will make the recipient feel the movement more.

Hip rotation

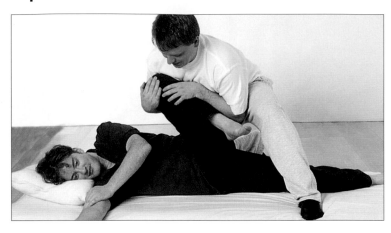

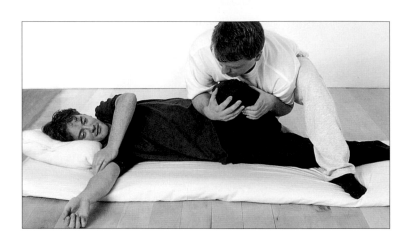

1. Lift the knee and hold it close to your body.

2. Then use your body to rotate the leg and move the hip.

Work the rest of the meridian
Keep the leg high, as this helps to expose the gall-bladder meridian.

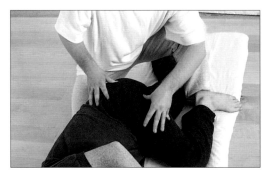

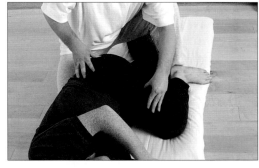

1. Work down the meridian in the side of the leg, beginning at the top.

2. Continue working along the meridian, down the leg.

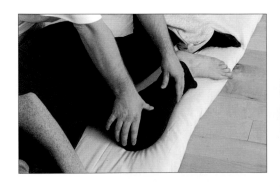

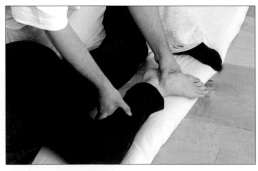

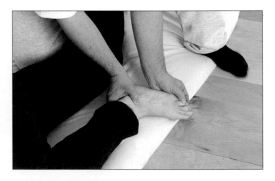

3. Work slowly and gently until you reach the end of the meridian.

4. Remember in particular to work gall-bladder point 34 (below the knee) and, as illustrated, gall-bladder point 40 (on the ankle crease).

5. Equally important is gall-bladder point 44, at the end of the fourth toe.

Work the liver meridian

Work along the exposed part of the liver meridian on the other leg.

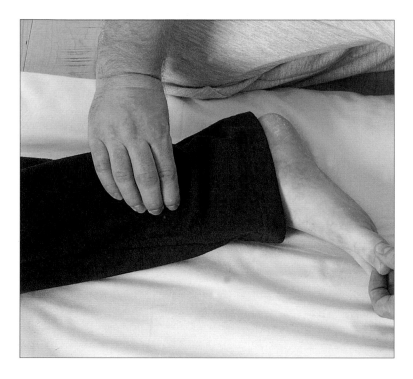

1. This starts at the big toe.

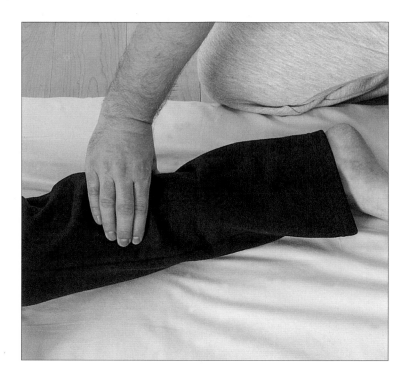

2. The meridian extends along the leg.

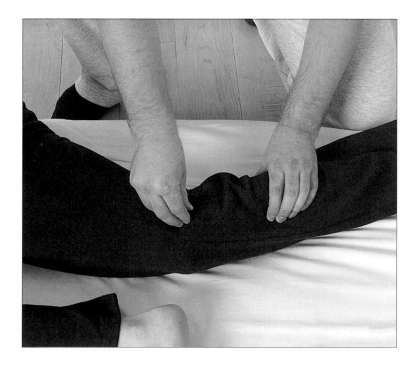

3. It goes through the groin area. Do not work as far up as the groin in a treatment session.

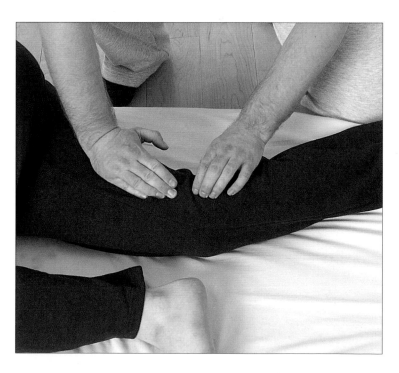

Ask your client to turn over so that you can work the other side of their body.

Working in the sitting position

Being treated in the sitting position is frequently people's first taste of Shiatsu, either as a brief treatment by a friend or at a demonstration. The fact that many decide to take further treatments or learn the art afterwards shows how effective a good treatment can be in the sitting position.

The recipient can be seated either on a chair or on the floor. If the recipient is on a chair, the shape of the chair may limit your movements, but it may well be more comfortable for the recipient. There is nothing to stop you from practising any treatment in the sitting position if you wish. The following is a simple treatment that you can normally perform in about fifteen minutes.

Palm the back	**Palm down the bladder meridian**	**Use thumbs into the bladder meridian**
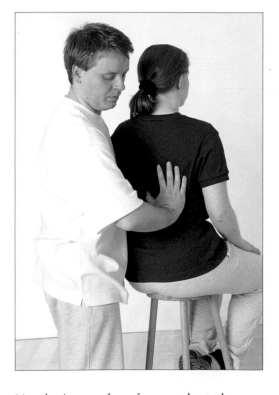	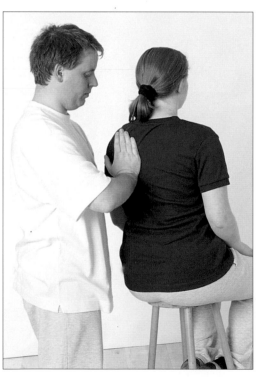	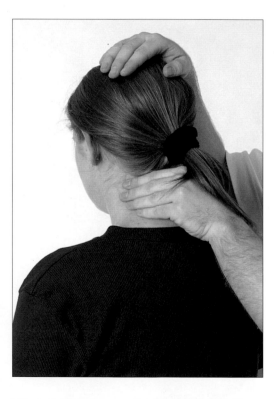
Use the inner edge of your palm to loosen the back.	Activate the bladder meridian by palming down it.	Work the Tsubos on the bladder meridian.

Loosen the neck

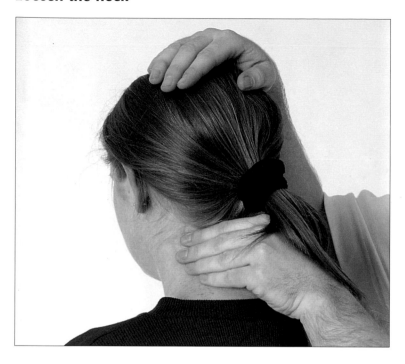

Give a general massage to the neck to loosen it.

Neck rotations

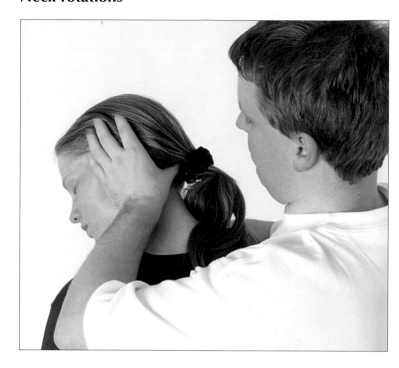

Place your finger and thumb into the occiput and gently work the neck through a half-circle (never a full circle).

Rotate the shoulder

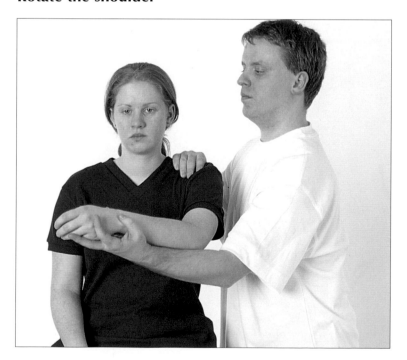

Hold the torso steady with one hand (try to get your fingers into some points that you know) and rotate the shoulder with your other hand.

Arm rotations

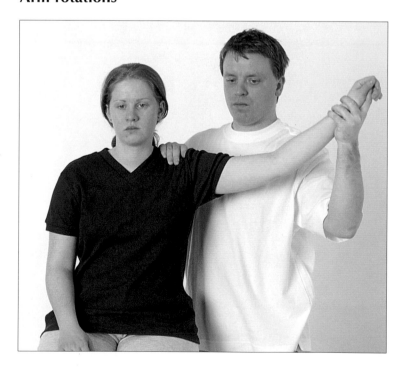

Hold the shoulder and wrist so that you can rotate the arm through a clockwise and anti-clockwise direction.

Massage down the arm

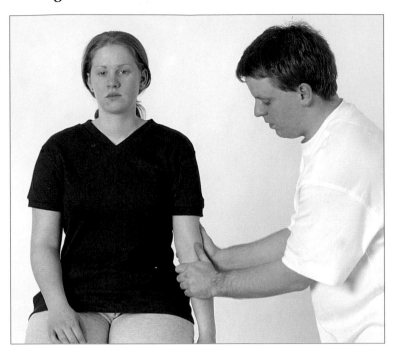

Gently loosen the muscles down the arm.

Work the wrist

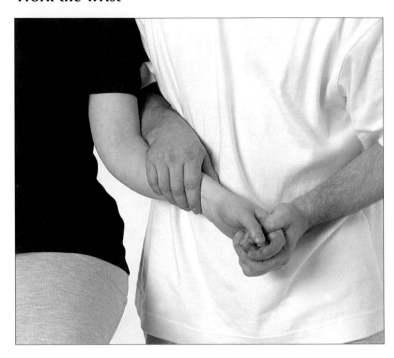

Rotate the wrist and loosen it.

Loosen the fingers

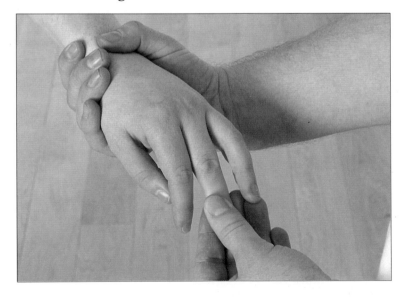

Rotate and massage all five fingers and the palm of the hand individually.

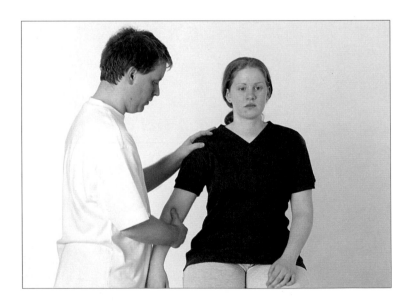

Repeat the procedure for the other arm.

Self-Shiatsu

If you want to learn the locations of the meridians, you will need to practise your art. A good way of practising is on yourself. This will both help you to absorb the information and is good for your health.

The name 'Do-In' is given to self-Shiatsu. There are some schools that teach Do-In as a core part of their lessons. It is worth working out a sequence that you can practise. You can use it as an invigorating start to the day or as a way of relaxing in the evening.

The following sequence contains useful techniques for Do-In and can be practised at any time of the day. It will take about ten minutes when you have learned the sequence.

Massage the crown of your head

The crown point is where all of the Yin meridians eventually meet up. Massage the point by rotating it gently with your fingertips. Bring intent from your fingertips down through your body.

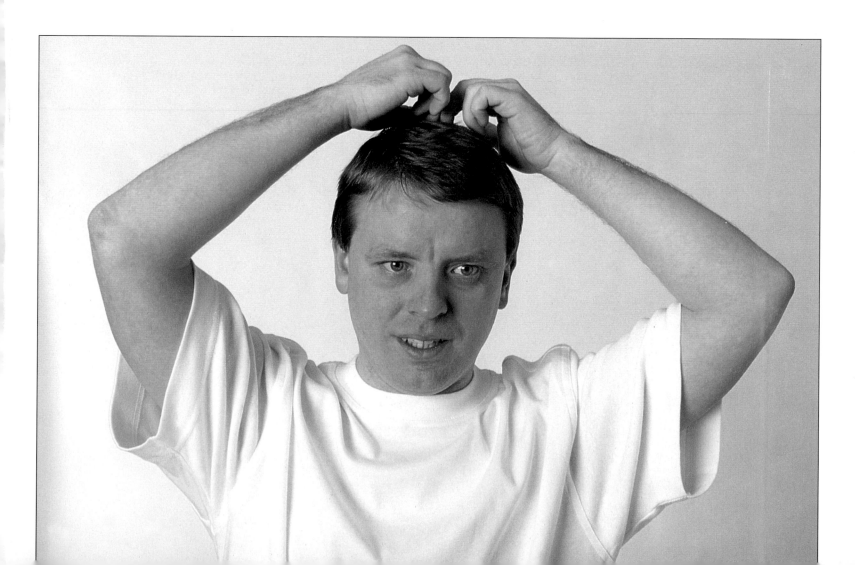

Chi facewash

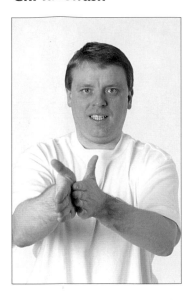 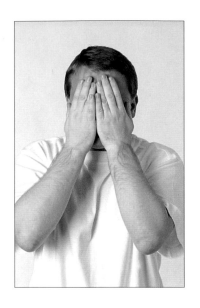 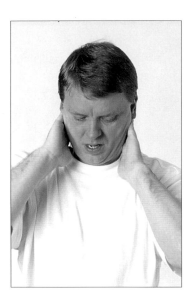 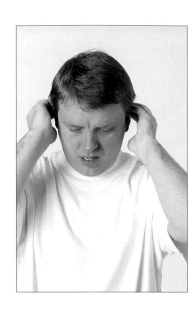

1. Rub your hands together until they are quite warm.

2. Rub your face and scalp with your warm hands as though you were washing them. When your hands cool down, warm them again by rubbing them.

3. Do not forget to wash behind your ears!

4. There are many points around the ear.

Tap the head and neck

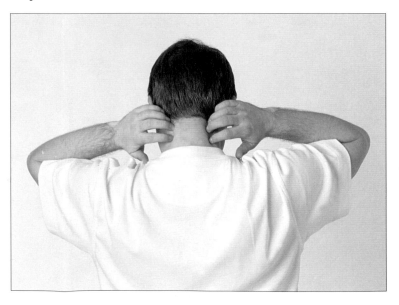 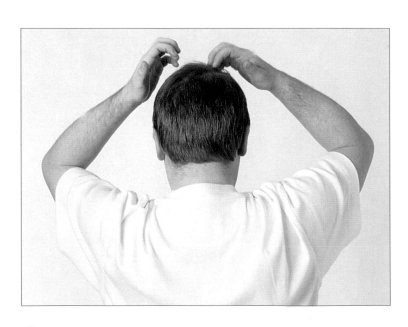

1. Keep your hands loose and tap your neck with the tips of your fingers.

2. Then move on and tap your scalp in the same way.

Opening the forehead

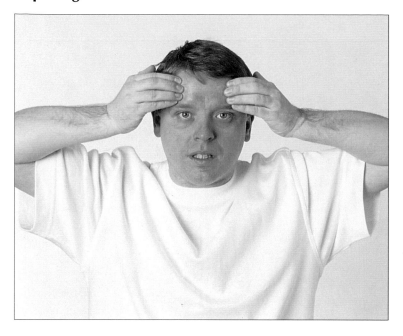

Use your fingertips to smooth across your forehead.

Opening the neck

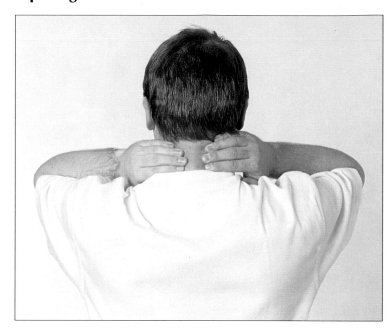

Use the same movement to open the back of the neck.

Neck rotation

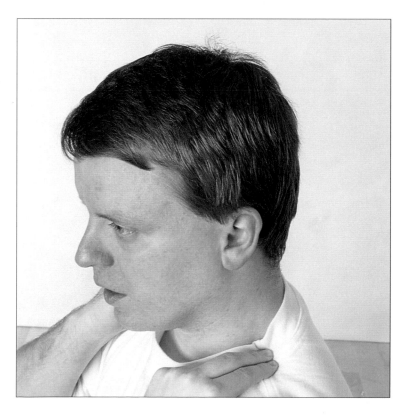

1. Place your fingers in gall-bladder point 21.

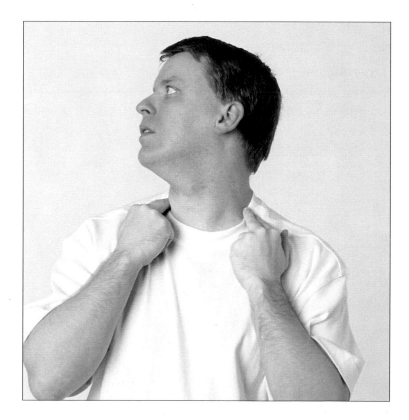

2. Then gently rotate your neck from side to side.

Tap your shoulder

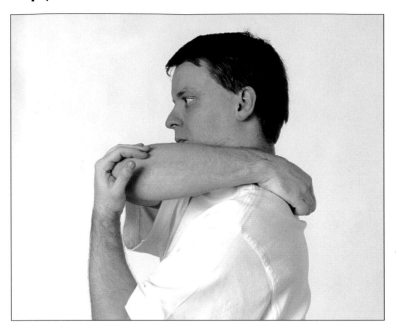

Make a loose fist with one hand and tap your shoulder and upper back. It may help to use your other hand to push your elbow and reach further.

Tap your inner arm

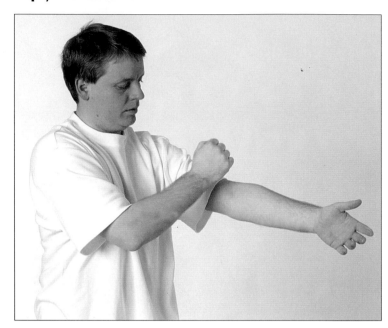

Tap along your inner arm. Try to tap along the lung, pericardium and heart meridians.

Tap your outer arm

Tap your outer arm, moving along the large-intestine, triple-heater and small-intestine meridians.

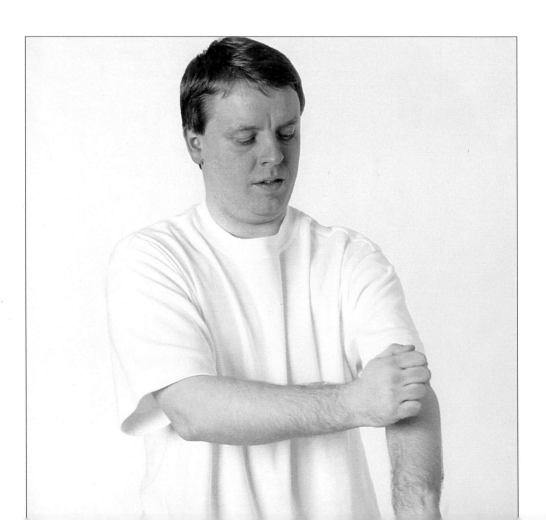

Tap your chest and abdomen

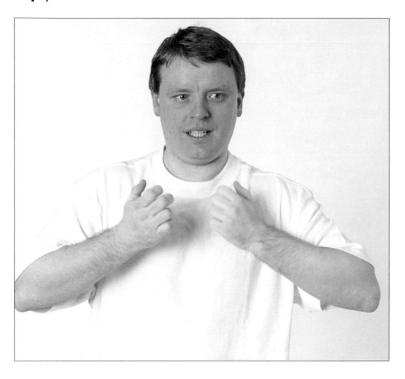

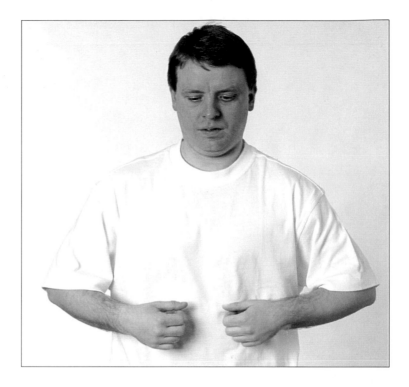

1. First use your fingertips or loose fists to tap the chest gently.

2. Then move your hands down and use the same procedure on your abdomen.

Tap your back

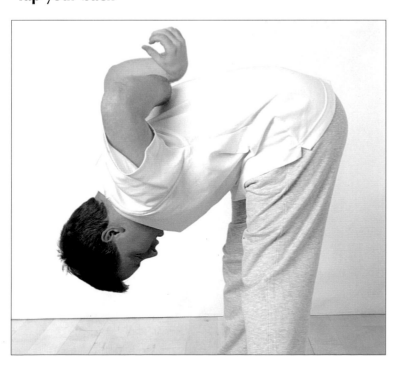

Tap your legs

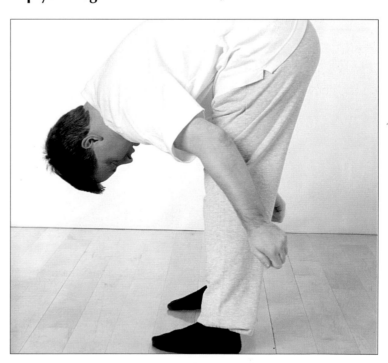

You will improve your range of movement if you bend forwards to tap your back. Pay attention to your sacrum and try to tap along the bladder meridian.

Tap down the Yang meridians (bladder, stomach and gall bladder) and up the Yin meridians (kidney, spleen and liver).

Massage your Hara

Spiral outwards from your navel, moving in a clockwise direction.

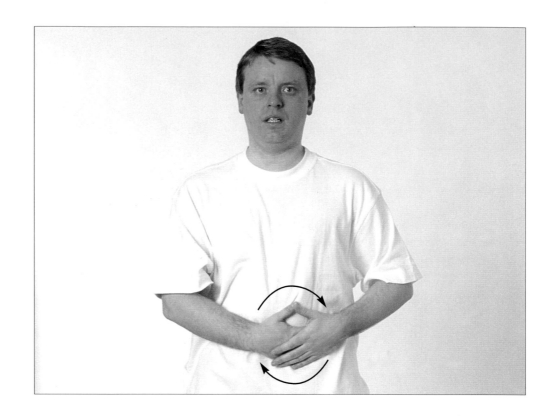

Massage your ankles, feet and toes

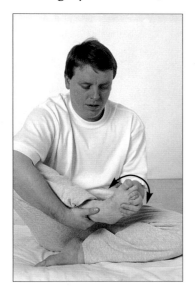 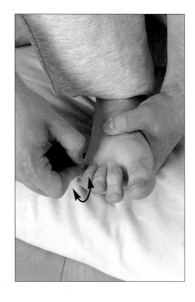 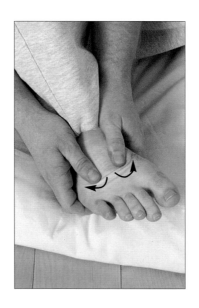 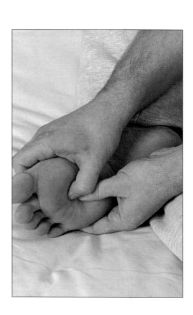

1. Sit down and rotate your ankles.

2. Then rotate each of your toes in turn.

3. Perform a general massage to loosen your feet.

4. Finish by massaging the start of the kidney meridian in the middle of your foot.

Typical Shiatsu procedures

The following list is not intended to be complete or unchangeable. It is simply a list of some examples of the use of Shiatsu. You may give a treatment that is quite different from the examples shown here, and it could still work perfectly. The best approach is to be sensitive to the person whom you are treating.

If you do have experience of treating an ailment, you should be mindful of it, but still stay in the present treatment that you are working on.

Acid stomach

Acid stomach is a common result of stress. Work the earth meridians in the feet to draw the energy downwards. Shiatsu to the Hara can be helpful. Here the practitioner is holding stomach points 42 and 45.

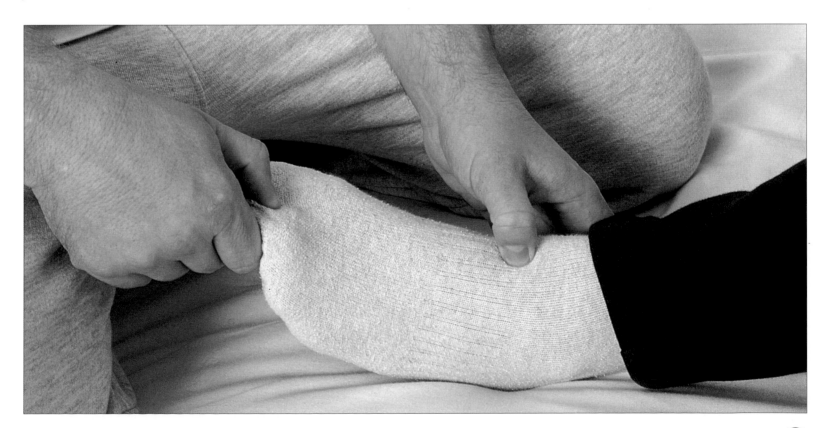

Allergies

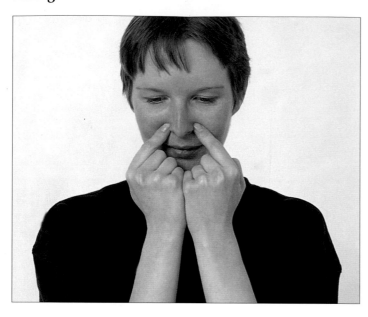

Allergies can sometimes show a weakness in the immune system. Work with the lungs, spleen and kidney to give strength to the immune system. Large-intestine point 20 is useful for calming sneezing. This is something that anyone can do for him- or herself.

Angina

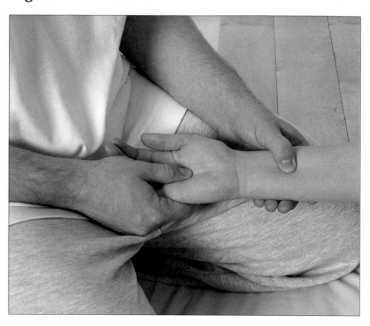

Use any of the fire-energy meridians. Here the practitioner is holding points 6 and 8 on the pericardium.

Anxiety

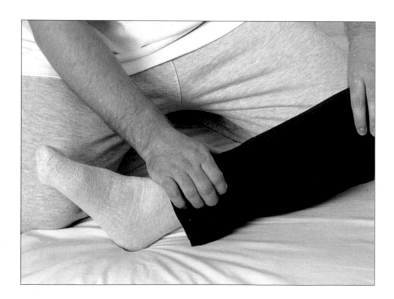

Worry and anxiety are typical examples of a weakness in the earth Ki. This can invade the water energy, causing fear and phobia. Here you see spleen points 6 and 9. Spleen point 9 is the water point.

Asthma

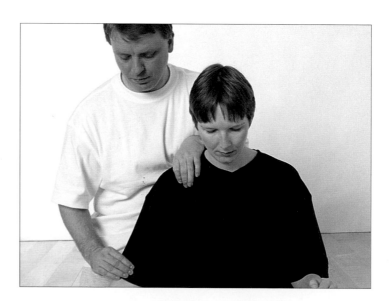

Asthma is caused by a weakness in the lungs and kidneys, therefore work with the metal and water elements may help. Here the practitioner works the lung meridian. Work the earth and water elements. If the mind needs calming, try the heart channel.

Cramp

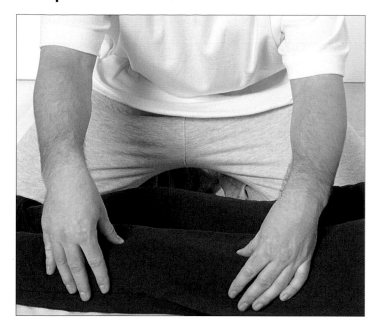

Work the bladder meridian behind, and below, the knee. Stretching is important to relieve cramp.

Constipation

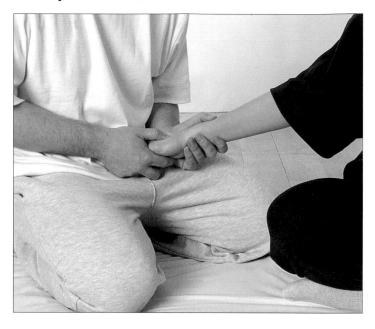

Hara work can help with the dispersal of the blocked energy. A deep, wave-like rocking may start the movement. Work the large-intestine meridian. Here point 4 is shown.

Diarrhoea

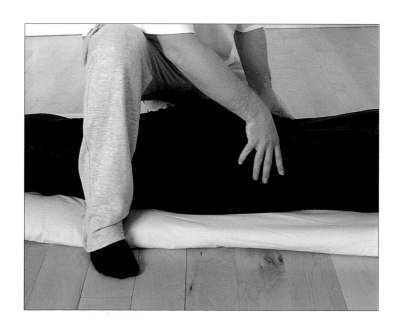

1. Treat the bladder and kidney meridians, paying particular attention to the large-intestine point on the bladder channel at bladder point 25.

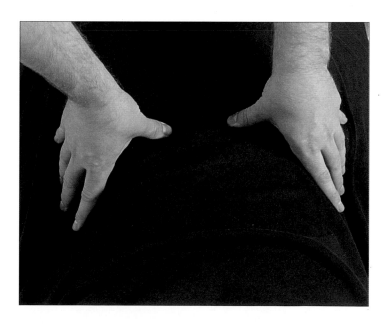

2. Bladder point 25 is at the top of the sacrum. Help the bowel function by treating the large-intestine meridian.

Earache

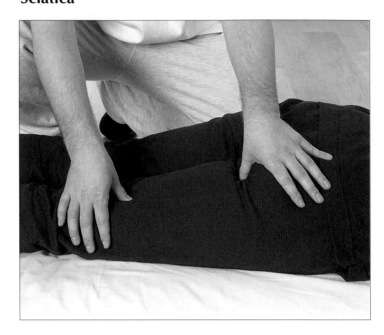

Treat any of the points around the ear. Pay special attention to the gall-bladder meridian because the wood element controls the ears.

Sciatica

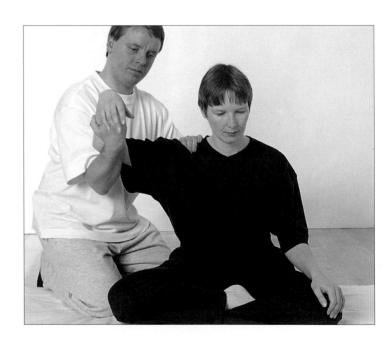

Gentle work along the bladder meridian is usually helpful.

Frozen shoulder

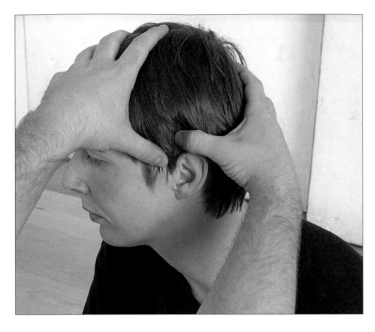

1. Work with points in, or around, the shoulder and tone any deficiencies. Here the practitioner is working on small-intestine points 10 and 11.

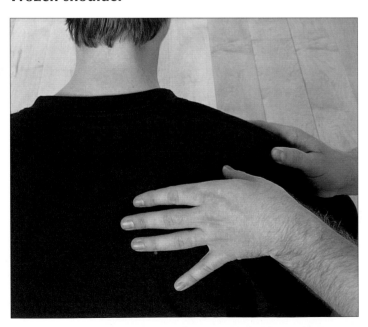

2. Mobilising techniques will be helpful.

When not to use Shiatsu

Shiatsu can be used to help a wide variety of illnesses and complaints. There are, however, a few cases where you should either not attempt a treatment or should refer your client to an expert. As a beginner, it is inadvisable to treat life-threatening conditions, such as heart disease or cancer.

Do not treat anybody who has a highly contagious disease or fever. In cases such as burns, breaks, cuts, open sores or varicose veins, it is best to avoid the injury site if you are attempting a treatment. It may simply aggravate the condition if you touch it. Avoid Hara work with women who have a contraceptive coil, as it will cause discomfort.

Pregnant women may find Shiatsu very helpful. As a beginner, there is very little that you could do that would cause harm to the mother or unborn baby.

However, there are some points that should not be used during pregnancy, as follows.

Large-intestine 4

Spleen 1 and 6

Gall-bladder 21

Liver 3

Bladder 60 and 67

Kidney 3

If you treat a pregnant woman, quickly revise these points before you begin.

Reflections on Shiatsu

Shiatsu is not a unique science that stands on its own. It comes from many rich sources of knowledge, some of which are in common use today.

Acupuncture is like a sister science to Shiatsu. The same meridians and points are used as in Shiatsu; the difference is that your therapist will use needles to work the points instead of thumbs. The treatment will be done on bare skin.

Some acupuncturists use a technique called 'cupping'. Cupping involves the use of a glass cup. A flame is placed inside the cup to evacuate the air. The cup is then placed on specific points and the vacuum inside the cup draws Ki to the surface.

Acupuncturists and Shiatsu therapists sometimes use Moxa. The most common method is to use a Moxa stick, which looks rather like a cigar. The burning end of the stick is placed near points to bring heat to the body.

Chi Gung healing is frequently taught by therapists to help the client to heal themselves. Some therapists use Chi Gung for giving treatments that work with the energy field of the body.

Martial arts and meditation are frequently used to help therapists and clients. Karate is also from Japan, and some karate masters teach Shiatsu, too. Tai Chi is an ideal complementary art to Shiatsu because it teaches you how to understand energy better and to work from your Hara.

Shiatsu evolves with time and location. If you were to receive a treatment in Japan, it would feel different from a treatment in the West. This need not be an issue because it simply means that the therapist has developed their energy in a different way, with a slightly different physiology to deal with.

Connection

One of the fundamental basics of Shiatsu is that you need to learn how to make a connection. Loss of connection with self or others causes suffering. Imagine yourself in solitary confinement for a period of time and you will probably not doubt the fact.

Conversely, try to imagine hurting a person with whom you feel a genuine sense of connection. A sense of connection helps you to create a link of empathy between yourself and others.

Connection with yourself is important before you can feel connection with others. A drug addict will not normally think too much about any damage that they are inflicting on themselves. Think about how many things you do to harm yourself before you judge the drug addict. If you drive too fast to work in the morning you risk not only injuring yourself, but others as well.

A violent person will not think about the pain and suffering that they are inflicting upon another person. A martial arts expert would never actually use their skill unless in an extreme situation. The difference is that the martial artist has been trained to respect themselves and others.

One of the greatest problems of our time is that we are destroying the planet that we live upon. Pollution and destruction are acts of violence that are directed towards the Earth rather than against an individual. The company that pours dangerous chemicals into a river has forgotten the fact that we need the Earth to live upon. By destroying our environment, we destroy a part of our own lives and of those that follow us.

In this sense, Shiatsu helps us to feel connected with ourselves, others and the universe as a whole. The very fact that touch is the central feature of the art is a physical aspect of this. Even the most cynical of the critics who dispute the fact that Shiatsu can be beneficial would not be able to argue against this. Shiatsu can therefore be seen as a way of improving our links with ourselves, others and the world we live in.

Glossary

Acupuncture: a healing art that uses needles to puncture the skin at certain points that have an effect on the rest of the body.

Anma: part of the roots of Shiatsu, a system that used the energy channels or meridians.

Cun: pronounced 'sun', the system of measurement used in Shiatsu.

Do-In: self-Shiatsu.

Energy: in this context, the basic life force of nature.

Five elements: a system based on observations of nature through its cycles.

Hara: the main reservoir of energy located in the abdomen.

Jing: the life force.

Karate: a Japanese martial art using fast, dynamic motion generated from the Hara.

Ki: the Japanese word for 'energy' (Chi in Chinese).

Ko cycle: the controlling, or destructive, cycle.

Kyo-Jitsu: 'empty and full', energetic qualities of Tsubo.

Macrobiotic Shiatsu: a branch of Shiatsu that emphasises dietary concepts.

Macrocosmic: the very large.

Makkaho stretches: a series of stretches designed to stretch pairs of meridians.

Meridian: the name given to the path, or channel, that the flow of energy takes.

Microcosmic: the very small.

Moxa: a herb (mugwort) that is burned to generate heat.

Qigong or Chi Gung: exercises designed specifically to work with the body's energetic system.

Sacrum: the bony part at thebottom of the spine.

Shen: consciousness.

Shen cycle: the nurturing, or creative, cycle.

Shiatsu: a healing art based on touch, Eastern techniques and philosophies.**Tai Chi:** a Chinese martial art based on self-defence, health and philosophy.

Tan Tien: an energy point at the centre of the Hara.

Tao: the great unnameable! A philosophy that observes nature and its rhythms.

Ten thousand things: the Taoist term for the many things in the universe (ten thousand was once thought to be a massive number).

Tsubo: a point that can be used to manipulate energy in a meridian.

Yang: the opposite of Yin. The male, or expanding, part of the cycle.

Yin: the opposite of Yang. The female, or receptive, part of the cycle.

Zen Shiatsu: a branch of Shiatsu that uses an extended meridian system.

Index

Acknowledgements

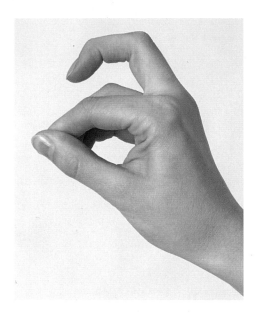

I would like to thank my wife, Carol, for her love and support during my training, and also for allowing me to practise my Shiatsu technique on her.

I would also like to thank Sue Hix and Tom Litten, of the Rosewell Shiatsu Centre in Castle Bytham, Lincolnshire, for their excellent teaching and their patience with me during that teaching. Finally, I would like to thank my brother Mark for his assistance with my understanding of some of the biological aspects of the art.

Picture credits

Image on page 19b © 2001 Photodisk, Inc.

Images on page 8, 12, 16l, 17, 18, 20, 21b, 23b, 26, 32b, 34b, 35b, 37b, 38b, 39b, 40b, 41b, 42, 44b, 45, 46, 66, 67, 68, 124 © Stockbyte.

(Where l = left, r = right, t = top and b = bottom.)